# IT HAPPENED TO ME

Series Editor: Arlene Hirschfelder

Books in the It Happened to Me series are designed for inquisitive teens digging for answers about certain illnesses, social issues, or lifestyle interests. Whether you are deep into your teen years or just entering them, these books are gold mines of up-to-date information, riveting teen views, and great visuals to help you figure out stuff. Besides special boxes highlighting singular facts, each book is enhanced with the latest reading lists, websites, and an index. Perfect for browsing, there are loads of expert information by acclaimed writers to help parents, guardians, and librarians understand teen illness, tough situations, and lifestyle choices.

1. *Epilepsy: The Ultimate Teen Guide,* by Kathlyn Gay and Sean McGarrahan, 2002.
2. *Stress Relief: The Ultimate Teen Guide,* by Mark Powell, 2002.
3. *Learning Disabilities: The Ultimate Teen Guide,* by Penny Hutchins Paquette and Cheryl Gerson Tuttle, 2003.
4. *Making Sexual Decisions: The Ultimate Teen Guide,* by L. Kris Gowen, 2003.
5. *Asthma: The Ultimate Teen Guide,* by Penny Hutchins Paquette, 2003.
6. *Cultural Diversity—Conflicts and Challenges: The Ultimate Teen Guide,* by Kathlyn Gay, 2003.
7. *Diabetes: The Ultimate Teen Guide,* by Katherine J. Moran, 2004.
8. *When Will I Stop Hurting? Teens, Loss, and Grief: The Ultimate Teen Guide to Dealing with Grief,* by Ed Myers, 2004.
9. *Volunteering: The Ultimate Teen Guide,* by Kathlyn Gay, 2004.
10. *Organ Transplants—A Survival Guide for the Entire Family: The Ultimate Teen Guide,* by Tina P. Schwartz, 2005.
11. *Medications: The Ultimate Teen Guide,* by Cheryl Gerson Tuttle, 2005.
12. *Image and Identity—Becoming the Person You Are: The Ultimate Teen Guide,* by L. Kris Gowen and Molly C. McKenna, 2005.
13. *Apprenticeship: The Ultimate Teen Guide,* by Penny Hutchins Paquette, 2005.
14. *Cystic Fibrosis: The Ultimate Teen Guide,* by Melanie Ann Apel, 2006.
15. *Religion and Spirituality in America: The Ultimate Teen Guide,* by Kathlyn Gay, 2006.

# EPILEPSY

## THE ULTIMATE TEEN GUIDE

### SECOND EDITION

### KATHLYN GAY

IT HAPPENED TO ME, NO. 52

ROWMAN & LITTLEFIELD
*Lanham • Boulder • New York • London*

Published by Rowman & Littlefield
A wholly owned subsidiary of The Rowman & Littlefield Publishing Group, Inc.
4501 Forbes Boulevard, Suite 200, Lanham, Maryland 20706
www.rowman.com

Unit A, Whitacre Mews, 26-34 Stannary Street, London SE11 4AB

British Library Cataloguing in Publication Information Available

**Library of Congress Cataloging-in-Publication Data**
Names: Gay, Kathlyn, author.
Title: Epilepsy : the ultimate teen guide / Kathlyn Gay.
Description: Second edition. | Lanham : Rowman & Littlefield, [2017] | Series: Happened to
    me ; no. 52 | Includes bibliographical references and index.
Identifiers: LCCN 2016035802 (print) | LCCN 2016037834 (ebook) | ISBN 9781442271715
    (hardback : alk. paper) | ISBN 9781442271722 (electronic)
Subjects: LCSH: Epilepsy in adolescence—Juvenile literature. | Epilepsy—Juvenile literature.
Classification: LCC RJ496.E6 G39 2017 (print) | LCC RJ496.E6 (ebook) | DDC
    616.85/300835—dc23
LC record available at https://lccn.loc.gov/2016035802

∞™ The paper used in this publication meets the minimum requirements of American
National Standard for Information Sciences—Permanence of Paper for Printed Library
Materials, ANSI/NISO Z39.48-1992.

Printed in the United States of America

# Contents

# Acknowledgments

My sincere thanks to Gillian Mangan for sharing her *Elegy to Epilepsy* and her upbeat online blog and to Dr. Kristin Seaborg for sharing her excerpt from her book *The Sacred Disease: A Memoir of Life with Epilepsy*. I am indebted also to all the people who have related their experiences with epileptic seizures through posts on various Internet media, in person, and in published materials.

My sincere thanks to Sean McGarrahan for sharing his experiences and Gillian Mangan for "An Elegy to Epilepsy" and her upbeat online blog. Also I thank Dr. Kristin Seaborg for sharing her excerpt from her book *The Sacred Disease: A Memoir of Life with Epilepsy*. I am indebted to all the people who have related their experiences with epileptic seizures through posts on various Internet media, in person, and in published materials.

# ABOUT EPILEPSY

*"When I'm about to have a seizure . . . I start to feel dizzy and my head hurts and or I feel nauseous."—teenager Kayla Brown*[1]

What *is* epilepsy? First, obviously, it's a noun. Second, it's the name of a neurological brain disorder. And third, it's a common condition that usually does not manifest itself until a seizure occurs. A person who has a seizure may experience uncontrollable muscle movements, violent shaking, froth, and blackout. Or the seizure may be mild with a person just staring into space or dropping her or his head. Seizures happen because of sudden, abnormal electrical activity in the brain.

Each year, an estimated 150,000 people, or 48 out of every 100,000 people will develop epilepsy. One in twenty-six people will have epilepsy at some time in their life, according to the Epilepsy Foundation.[2] "Epilepsy affects more people than multiple sclerosis, cerebral palsy, muscular dystrophy and Parkinson's combined," states Citizens United for Research in Epilepsy (CURE).[3]

Although such statistics may seem daunting, numerous individuals with epilepsy have led productive lives. A person with epilepsy could be a computer specialist, a professor, an author, a physicist, a musician, or an accomplished individual in other fields. The same is true for adolescents and teenagers with epilepsy, who may be outstanding students or champion athletes or community activists.

Yet young people with epilepsy seldom want others outside their families and close friends to know about their disorder, especially after the initial diagnosis. Why? Because epilepsy carries a stigma, which is the result of myths, misinformation, and misconceptions about the condition that have prevailed for thousands of years, and unfortunately are still widespread.

A teenager who calls herself Angel Princess Maria explained on the Epilepsy Foundation's Teen Zone forum in 2016:

There's been some times when I feel like I am not wanted [in] places because of my seizures. . . . I mean do they just hate me because I have seizures and they just don't know what to do to help me because I have a seizure. . . . I don't think it is fair for people to do this because aren't we just like all of them but with seizures in our life. . . . Times like this makes you think that your life sucks a lot.[4]

Some teens also are afraid that if they have a seizure they will be seen as weird, crazy, mentally disabled, or contagious. None of these assumptions are true. Another concern is about "hovering"—that is, school personnel or a supervisor at a part-time job will force a person who has had a seizure to go home even though his or her symptoms are gone. However, "The more people are involved and are educated about what [epilepsy] is, they won't be so worried [about epileptic seizures]," said an anonymous teenager on YouTube.[5]

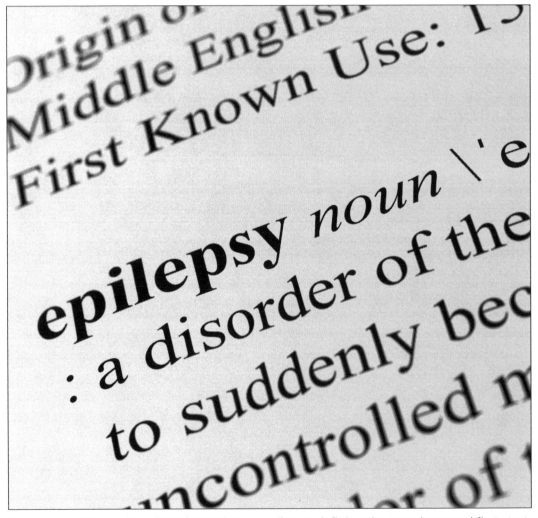

For young adults looking for information on epilepsy, defining the term is a good first start.
©iStock/Andrey Prokhorov

When diagnosed with epilepsy, some young people say they feel as though their life is about to end or that they will suffer mental impairment from an epileptic seizure. Or they fear that they will become outcasts—that their peers will avoid them. Some may become depressed, extremely angry, or defiant.

Kayla Brown was a high school honor student with a 3.48 grade point average when she told her story for WebMD. She wrote that she had her first seizure when she was five years old. She learned later that she had

a "petit mal" seizure or an "absence" seizure. It's called that because there's a lapse in conscious activity for a couple of seconds. It's different from a "grand mal" seizure, when people have convulsions. Once the doctor diagnosed me after that first seizure, we were able to learn about the disease and how to manage it. For instance, I take antiseizure medication

## Successful People with Epilepsy

Some people with epilepsy have become highly successful. They include Prince, the late singer/performer; Rick Harrison, star of TV's reality show *Pawn Stars*; Danny Glover, actor and multiple Emmy nominee; Jason Snelling, former Atlanta Falcons running back; Neil Young, Canadian rock star; Mighty Mike of the Harlem Wizards basketball team; and Chanda Gunn, the goalie for the 2006 women's U.S. Olympic ice hockey team.

Dozens of famous people from the past are often cited in lectures and articles online as having epileptic seizures. However, Dr. John R. Hughes of the University of Illinois at Chicago Medical School conducted a study of forty-three famous historic individuals from Pythagoras to Richard Burton. Hughes investigated records of such individuals as Aristotle, Leonardo da Vinci, Sir Isaac Newton, William Pitt, James Madison, Edgar Allen Poe, Agatha Christie, and Truman Capote—all of whom supposedly had epileptic seizures. But he found that none of the individuals studied had the disorder. Instead they had problems such as anxiety, alcohol and drug withdrawal, religious hallucinations, intense fear, and angst. Hughes noted that his "attempt to correct the record with respect to these people" was a reminder that "similar misdiagnoses are being made today."[a]

daily, and that keeps my seizures under control. But I still get them some-times, such as when I get dehydrated or stressed, or my medication level falls too low. I can tell when I'm about to have a seizure because I start to feel dizzy and my head hurts or I feel nauseous. If that happens, I tell an adult that I'm about to have a seizure. Afterward, I check in with my pediatrician and my neurologist just to make sure everything's OK.[6]

## Epileptic Seizures

Epileptic seizures cannot be defined as a single set of symptoms with specific characteristics. They affect people in diverse ways. When there is sudden, abnormal electrical activity in the brain, a person will likely have a seizure. "When people think of seizures, they often think of convulsions in which a person's body shakes rapidly and uncontrollably. Not all seizures cause convulsions. There are many types of seizures and some have mild symptoms," according to the U.S. National Library of Medicine. "Most seizures last from 30 seconds to 2 minutes and do not cause lasting harm. However, it is a medical emergency if seizures last longer than 5 minutes or if a person has many seizures and does not wake up between them."[7]

There are two main groups of seizures: focal, or partial, seizures and generalized seizures. An explanation on KidsHealth.com, which was reviewed by Harry S. Abram, MD, explains seizures this way:

> Partial seizures start in one part of the brain. The electrical disturbances may then move to other parts of the brain or they may stay in one area until the seizure is over. A person having a partial seizure may lose consciousness. There may be twitching of a finger or several fingers, a hand or arm, or a leg or foot. Certain facial muscles might twitch. Speech might become slurred, unclear, or unusual during the seizure. . . . It all depends on where in the brain the abnormal electrical activity is taking place.
>
> Generalized seizures involve electrical disturbances that occur all over the brain at the same time. The person may appear to be daydreaming, may stare off into space, or may pass out. The muscles may stiffen and the person might make sudden jerking motions, such as flinging the arms outward. He or she may suddenly go limp and slump down or fall over.[8]

### Atonic Seizures

One type of seizure that also may cause a person to fall is an atonic seizure in which a person's muscles become weak. A person's head may drop or he or she

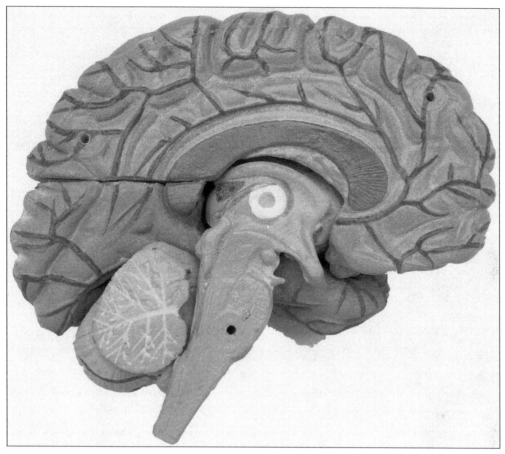

Anatomical model of human brain.

may fall but usually remain conscious. "These seizures usually last less than 15 seconds," according to the Epilepsy Foundation. "Because atonic seizures are so abrupt, without any warning, and because the people who experience them fall with force, atonic seizures can result in injuries to the head and face." Unless there are injuries, no first aid is needed.[9]

## What's a Brain?

Because the nature of a seizure depends on where it originates in the brain, it is important to know something about its parts and how it operates. A brain weighs less than three pounds and looks like a wrinkled walnut. It has the texture of thick jelly or gelatin, and is part of the central nervous system. It is what makes each person unique and is involved in emotions, thoughts, memory, sensations, dreams, and the control of movements.

Inside the brain is the cerebrum, the largest and most highly developed part of the human brain; it sits at the topmost part of the brain and is the source of intellectual activities and memories. The main parts of the brain are the right and left cerebral hemispheres and the brain stem. The two hemispheres are connected in the middle. An outer layer of the brain is gray matter made up of nerve cell bodies. Its inner layer is white matter comprised of insulated nerve fibers.

Each hemisphere of the brain's two hemispheres has four lobes: frontal, temporal, parietal, and occipital. Each of these lobes has different functions. The two frontal lobes lie directly behind the forehead. The frontal lobes affect movement, with the right frontal lobe involved in movement on a person's left side and just the opposite for the left frontal lobe. An injury to the left frontal lobe, for example, can cause motor impairment on the right side. At the rear of each frontal lobe is an area that helps control voluntary movement. A nearby place on the left frontal lobe is called Broca's area, which allows thoughts to be transformed into words. The frontal lobes help produce speech and make decisions.

The two sections behind the frontal lobes are called the parietal and occipital lobes. The parietal lobes interpret sensation such as touch and spatial perception. The occipital lobes are at the back of the brain and are involved in vision.

The functions of the temporal lobes are not as well understood as those of the other lobes, but the temporal lobes are responsible for distinguishing various sounds, tastes, and smells. They also help maintain balance and form memories. When temporal lobe seizures occur repeatedly over time, the hippocampus may be affected. The hippocampus is an area at the base of the brain that plays a role in one's memory and has been compared to the RAM of a computer. It stores data for a short time until it becomes part of the brain's long-term memory. The hippocampus can be damaged by repeated seizures.[10]

## Brain Cells

Whatever a person does—whether walking to class or hitting a baseball or reading a book—relies on neurons in brain cells that communicate with one another through electrical impulses and chemical signals carrying messages across different parts of the brain and between the brain and the rest of the nervous system. The human brain contains about 100 billion microscopic units called neurons, or nerve cells. Each nerve cell can produce and transmit electrical signals, and all are linked together in a complex network that allows the brain to do its work. Although nerve cells do not touch each other, one neuron can communicate with or stimulate another through an electrical-chemical process. Electrical impulses or signals begin "firing" or discharging to send messages. ("Electrical signals" are not actually electric because ions travel down the axon, not electrons. For the sake of simplicity, specialists use the term *electrical*.) An impulse travels from one cell to another through *axons* and *dendrites* (from the Greek word *dendron*, meaning "tree").

Axons are cable-like structures that carry information away from a cell, and dendrites are like tiny tentacles that receive and deliver signals. Chemicals called neurotransmitters direct electrical impulses across a gap, known as a *synapse,* between nerve cells. The receiving cell has receptors that are activated and can "excite" or inhibit the neuron. If the nerve cell is excited (or stimulated), it fires a signal and the process continues. If neurotransmitters inhibit a neuron, they do not fire or send a signal. When the brain functions properly, there is a balance between excitement and inhibition.

Axons may be very short, such as those that carry signals from one cell in the cortex to another cell less than a hair's width away. Or axons may be very long, such as those that carry messages from the brain all the way down the spinal cord.

When the signal reaches the end of the axon it stimulates tiny sacs that release chemicals known as neurotransmitters into the synapse. The neurotransmitters cross the synapse and attach to receptors on the neighboring cell. These receptors can change the properties of the receiving cell. If the receiving cell is also a neuron, the signal can continue the transmission to the next cell.

## Nonepileptic Seizures

Seizures that are not related to a physical brain disorder are medically known as nonepileptic seizures (NES) or events. An NES may appear to be like an epileptic seizure, but is not the result of abnormal electrical discharges. Often nonepileptic events are related to stress or emotional traumas and are known as psychogenic nonepileptic seizures (PNES).

According to Phylis Feiner Johnson, who has epilepsy, "Because symptoms of these disorders can look very much like epileptic seizures, they are often mistaken for epilepsy. Distinguishing between true epileptic seizures and nonepileptic events can be very difficult and requires a thorough medical assessment, careful monitoring, and knowledgeable health professionals."[11]

A study published in Elsevier's *Seizure Journal* in 2012 revealed that many patients admitted to the Johns Hopkins epilepsy unit did not have the disorder; rather they had nonepileptic seizures. The study concluded that "patients with PNES report more distress associated with negative life events than do neurologically normal individuals and patients with epilepsy." When patients with PNES are misdiagnosed, they may spend years being treated with epilepsy medications that are ineffective. If patients are diagnosed correctly with PNES, their symptoms simply disappear or they may receive psychiatric treatment and/or medications for anxiety and stress.[12]

Some instances of PNES may occur because of trauma such as "physical or sexual abuse, incest, divorce, death of a loved one, or other great loss or sudden

## How Brain Cells Work

The National Institute of Neurological Disorders and Stroke (NINDS) describes brain cells on the agency's website, which includes keys to graphics that show specific parts of the brain. These can be accessed at http://www.ninds.nih.gov/disorders/brain_basics/know_your_brain.htm. The NINDS explanation follows:

> The brain and the rest of the nervous system are composed of many different types of cells, but the primary functional unit is a cell called the neuron. . . . Neurons consist of three parts. The cell body . . . contains the nucleus, where most of the molecules that the neuron needs to survive and function are manufactured. Dendrites . . . extend out from the cell body like the branches of a tree and receive messages from other nerve cells. Signals then pass from the dendrites through the cell body and may travel away from the cell body down an axon . . . to another neuron, a muscle cell, or cells in some other organ. The neuron is usually surrounded by many support cells. Some types of cells wrap around the axon to form an insulating sheath. . . . This sheath can include a fatty molecule called myelin, which provides insulation for the axon and helps nerve signals travel faster and farther. Axons may be very short, such as those that carry signals from one cell in the cortex to another cell less than a hair's width away. Or axons may be very long, such as those that carry messages from the brain all the way down the spinal cord.
>
> Scientists have learned a great deal about neurons by studying the synapse—the place where a signal passes from the neuron to another cell. When the signal reaches the end of the axon it stimulates the release of tiny sacs. . . . These sacs release chemicals known as neurotransmitters . . . into the synapse. . . . The neurotransmitters cross the synapse and attach to receptors . . . on the neighboring cell. These receptors can change the properties of the receiving cell. If the receiving cell is also a neuron, the signal can continue the transmission to the next cell.[b]

change," according to the Epilepsy Foundation. "The most reliable test to make the diagnosis of PNES is EEG-video monitoring. During a video-EEG, the patient is monitored (over a time-period spanning anywhere from several hours to several days) with both a video camera and an EEG until a seizure occurs. Through analysis of the video and EEG recordings, the diagnosis of PNES can be made with near certainty. Upon diagnosis, the patient will usually be referred to a psychiatrist for further care."[13]

NES may also occur because someone has previously had a stroke. That was the case for Garrison Keillor, host of the famed *Prairie Home Companion.* On Memorial Day weekend in 2016, he suffered a seizure after a performance in Vienna, Virginia. Keillor told CNN news, "[After the show, I] flew to Mayo [in Minnesota] to get checked out and saw an MRI image of my skull with a black hole where a previous stroke struck close to the language center of the brain, so I came away feeling vastly fortunate." CNN reported that Keillor had had a previous seizure during 2016, but he was taking an anticonvulsant. He retired after forty years of his radio show in July 2016.[14]

Veterans also are at risk of NES/PNES or may suffer from the condition. Research has shown, however, that PNES may be misdiagnosed. "Veterans with psychogenic seizures were often four times more likely than civilians to be given seizure medications designed to treat epilepsy until a correct diagnosis was made," according to a 2011 WebMD report. In a study published in *Neurology*, "researchers reviewed the medical records of 203 veterans and 726 civilians who were admitted to an epilepsy monitoring unit over a 10-year period. During this time, 50 veterans were diagnosed with psychogenic seizures."[15] Currently, more research is being conducted to distinguish between epileptic seizures and nonepileptic events in veterans as well as civilians.

# FACTS AND MYTHS

*"Epilepsy stigma has been around as long as the condition itself.
I've even found examples . . . where people with epilepsy are described as being
possessed by demons, unclean, or sinners. We are far from that time now. . . .
But stigma is still around. And for me, the stigma surrounding epilepsy is worse than
the epilepsy itself."—anonymous young woman posting on GirlswithNerve.com[1]*

Throughout the ages, people have described epilepsy in hundreds of different ways. Ancient accounts on Babylonian tablets, for example, date as far back as 2000 BCE and describe many types of seizures. Babylonians were convinced that epileptic seizures were related to the supernatural and each type of seizure was named for a god or spirit. The ancient Greeks carried on this belief and associated epilepsy with the spiritual, calling it "the sacred disease."

It was also believed that the moon god Selene was responsible for epilepsy, and people with epilepsy were thought to be moonstruck, or *lunatic* (the Latin version of *moonstruck*). Treatment ranged from eating mistletoe to drinking dog urine to purges and bloodletting. The idea was to rid the body of evil spirits.

During the fifth century BC, the Greek medical scientist Hippocrates attempted to debunk beliefs about the spiritual nature of illnesses. In a collection of writings called the *Hippocratic Corpus*, Hippocrates and his followers argued against the idea that various diseases and disorders were caused by the gods. Hippocrates taught that epilepsy was a brain disorder, but his teachings did not dispel the widespread belief that people with epilepsy were possessed with demons.

Ancient Romans continued to believe in demon possession and thought epilepsy was contagious. Anyone who touched someone with epilepsy, it was believed, could be taken over by an evil spirit. A variety of magical practices were thought to provide protection, such as avoiding certain foods, wearing black clothing, and taking baths. Drinking human blood was also considered a protective measure—a way for a person with epilepsy to prevent a seizure.

To determine who had epilepsy, or the "falling sickness" as it was called, ancient Romans had a person suspected of the disorder smell a piece of jet, a stone or rock similar to coal. "If the person did not fall to the ground on smelling the stone, he was considered to be 'free of the falling sickness,'" according to the Epilepsy Museum in Germany. The museum noted,

> A similar test was undertaken using a potter's wheel. It was believed that a person with epilepsy would fall to the ground on watching the wheel turn. It is possible that people who actually did fall to the ground during this test actually did so as a result of their photosensibility. Flashing lights or glittering surfaces can trigger epileptic seizures in some people.[2]

## Driving Out Demons

During the early Christian era, epilepsy was still considered the work of evil spirits who possessed individuals. In Europe during the Middle Ages, the idea of demon possession continued. But medieval Christians believed that prayers

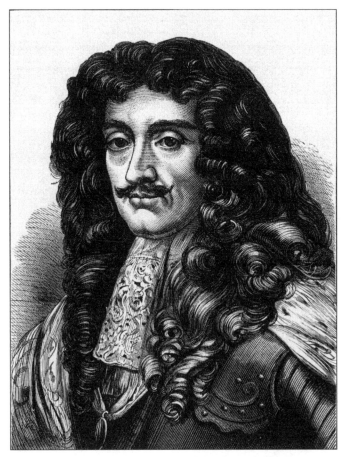

In 1685, King Charles II had a seizure and physicians shaved all the hair from his head in order to apply blistering agents to his scalp. The treatment did not work.

and sacred objects would protect against epilepsy or cure seizures. People fasted, made pilgrimages to sacred places, and called on saints, who were thought to have the power to intercede on behalf of someone with epilepsy. One of the most popular saints was Valentine of Germany. People seeking cures visited places where St. Valentine supposedly lived, and at one site in Alcase a hospital for epileptics was built during the fifteenth century. Since medieval times St. Valentine has been considered the patron saint of epilepsy.

For centuries, people with epilepsy not only suffered because of their disorder but also because of maltreatment by society at large. It was common to shun people who had seizures, isolating them in hospitals or other institutions because of fears that epilepsy was contagious. Punishment was another common treatment, especially when epilepsy was associated with witchcraft or the devil's work. Some people with epilepsy were thought to be witches and were burned at the stake.

Even royalty suffered brutal treatment. Consider King Charles II of England who had a seizure in 1685 while he was being shaved. At least a dozen physicians cared for him, but their treatments would hardly be called humane by today's standards. Doctors tried to purge his body by bloodletting, forcing him to vomit, administering enemas and laxatives repeatedly, and applying plasters made of

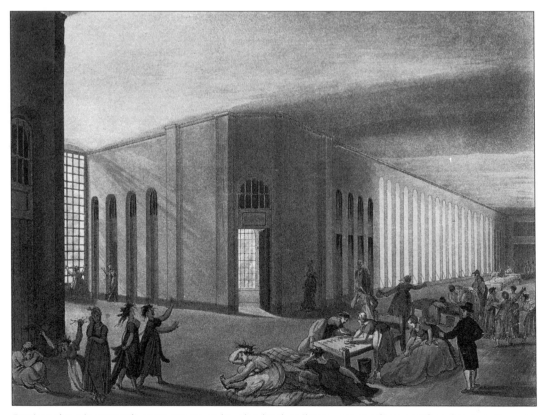

During the nineteenth century, people who had epilepsy were often confined in lunatic asylums, similar to the graphic shown here.

pigeon dung to his feet. The king's head was also shaved so that blistering agents could be applied to his scalp. The king did not improve, so he was given concoctions that included numerous herbs, extracts from a human skull, and ammonia water. Nothing helped. King Charles II died within two days, no doubt due in part to his treatments.

## Epilepsy Treatment in the 1800s and Early 1900s

During the early nineteenth century, people who had frequent and/or prolonged epileptic seizures and could not be cared for by family members were sometimes institutionalized in prisons, in asylums for the mentally handicapped or insane, or in places that once housed people with leprosy. In Belgium during the nineteenth century, psychiatric hospitals put epileptics in padded cage beds.

In the United States, the Minnesota legislature in 1909 created a department for incurables—that is, people considered "feeble-minded" or insane, the deaf and blind, and people with epilepsy. The incurables were institutionalized in a complex of about sixty buildings on 860 acres. At the time there were 210 people in the epileptic colony, as it was called, who were housed in five cottages. Minnesota lawmakers declared that the institution provided a home life for the feeble-minded and epileptics who could not live independently.[3]

Virginia passed a Eugenical Sterilization Act in 1924 requiring that people with epilepsy who were deemed "defective" and institutionalized had to be sterilized. Virginia was among more than thirty states that passed such laws. Celia Vandegrift, who once worked at the Lynchburg State Colony for Epileptics and Feebleminded, told *America Tonight* in 2014, "It's what our legislators wanted at the time and what our bosses wanted, even the President of the United States." Vandegrift was in her eighties when she spoke publicly for the first time about her involvement in one of America's leading eugenics programs. "You trusted all those people, so I went right along with them." She added, "I thought, at the time, I was doing the right thing. I can see now that it was so wrong." According to *America Tonight*'s report, "Virginia's 1924 Eugenical Sterilization Act [was] found constitutional by the Supreme Court three years later. . . . Officials estimate that 7,325 Virginians were sterilized under the law, which remained on the books until 1979. Approximately 65,000 forced sterilizations were conducted nationwide."[4]

A more humane concept developed when a London neurologist, John Hughlings Jackson, presented his theory that seizures (which at that time were called "fits") were caused by "occasional, sudden, excessive, rapid, and local discharges of grey matter."[5] Dr. Jackson also found that particular parts of the brain control specific parts of the body. Thus, he concluded, the characteristics of a seizure depend on where discharges take place in the brain. Today one type of seizure, which begins with a twitch in the toe or thumb and spreads to the leg or arm, leading to a convulsion, is called the Jacksonian march or Jacksonian seizure. Jackson's theories helped counteract the myth that epilepsy was a form of insanity and led to other theories and neurological discoveries.

In the 1920s Hans Berger, a German psychiatrist, developed the electroencephalogram (EEG), a test that reveals electrical discharges in the brain. The EEG confirmed the earlier Jackson assumptions and showed that the patterns of brainwave discharges vary with different types of seizures. With the EEG test, doctors were also able to locate where discharges originated.

## Cultural Beliefs about Epilepsy

In some areas of the world, including the United States, various cultural groups hold long-standing folk beliefs about epilepsy. For example, traditional Hmong, who have emigrated to the United States, have maintained their belief that epilepsy "is caused by a malevolent spirit called a dab, who captures someone's soul and makes him or her sick," according to author Anne Fadiman who wrote *The Spirit Catches You and You Fall Down* (Farrar, Straus and Giroux, 1997). Her comment was part of an interview conducted by the Epilepsy Foundation. Fadiman explained further that among traditional Hmong, "epilepsy is recognized as a serious illness that can cause great suffering, but it is also seen as a distinguished affliction, since (as in many cultures) Hmong epileptics often grow up to become shamans. . . . Seizures are viewed as an altered state, a potential point of entry into the spiritual realm to which the rest of us are denied access."[6]

Traditional cultural beliefs also prevail in parts of Africa. One study published in *Epilepsia* found that some Nigerians believe epilepsy is inherited or caused by witchcraft or brain damage. In addition, "epileptic persons suffer untold social deprivations and discrimination in education, employment, housing, marital life, etc."[7]

In the book *Hand Trembling, Frenzy Witchcraft, and Moth Madness: A Study of Navajo Seizure Disorders*, authors Jerrold E. Levy, Raymond Neutra, and Dennis Parker describe research efforts in five Native American communities (Navaho, Apache, Zuni, Tewas, and Hopis). The authors write that the Native American "terms denoting specific causes" are translated by the authors as "moth madness, frenzy witchcraft, and hand trembling. . . . Moth madness indicates that incest has taken place." Frenzy witchcraft "refers to sexual excess of women" (rarely men), while trembling is believed to be caused by a Gila monster.[8]

Folk cures for epilepsy also were popular among the general public in the United States during the twentieth century. Screen and TV star Danny Glover says his grandmother, who was convinced that someone had put a hex on Glover,

## Patent Medicine "Cure"

In the late 1800s, a pump maker by the name of Henry Root of Ohio called himself a doctor and sold patent medicines (nonprescription drugs). Root advertised a "cure" for epilepsy in newspapers across the United States and other countries such as Great Britain, Australia, and New Zealand. One of Root's ads stated,

I CURE FITS! When I say CURE I do not mean merely to stop them for a time, and then have them return again. I MEAN A RADICAL CURE. I have made the disease of FITS, EPILEPSY or FALLING SICKNESS, A life-long study. I WARRANT my remedy to CURE the worst cases. Because others have failed is no reason for not now receiving a cure. Send at once for a treatise and a FREE BOTTLE of my INFALLIBLE REMEDY.

Apparently Root's business did not thrive. He sold it and went back to making pumps.[a]

insisted that he drink glass after glass of grape juice to cure his seizures. From the time he was first diagnosed with epilepsy at the age of fifteen, he knew when it was going to happen. He would hear an excruciating noise, which was an aura or warning sign.

"Eventually, I could recognize it happening. Then I could say, wherever I was, 'Something is happening to me. Please grab me. Please hold me. I'm about to have a seizure,'" Glover wrote in a 2009 blog post on SharingMiracle.net, which was a thirty-minute public affairs television program.[9] At the age of thirty-five Glover's seizures stopped for some unknown reason. Now in his sixties, Glover is still healthy and an active supporter of the Epilepsy Foundation.

## Qs and As about Epilepsy

The following are typical questions about epilepsy that many people ask. Answers provided here are my adaptations from numerous print and electronic sources.

## Watch This!

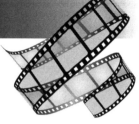

*SEIZED: Inside the Mystery of Epilepsy* is a Public Broadcasting System (PBS) documentary that tells and depicts
stories of children and young people with epilepsy. *SEIZED*
premiered in May 2016 and is an effort to bring epilepsy out in the open and
dispel the stigma surrounding it. Personal struggles of four individuals and their
families are shown along with comments from physicians. Some of the scenes
are difficult to watch as individuals have multiple seizures. Two of the patients in
the film are treated with cannabis oil, and one shows some progress in diminish-
ing seizures while the other does not. In addition, an army veteran who fought in
Afghanistan tells of his struggles with epilepsy that apparently are the result of
a brain injury during battle. He has had little success with treatment and has not
been able to get a job. The one-hour documentary is available at http://www.pbs
.org/program/seized-inside-mystery-epilepsy/.

*Q. Can a person inherit epilepsy?*

A. Some rare forms of epilepsy are inherited, and some people might have
a genetic makeup that leads to epileptic seizures. But most epilepsies
are not inherited.

*Q. Is epilepsy contagious?*

A. Absolutely not.

*Q. Is epilepsy a psychological problem?*

A. No.

*Q. Can epilepsy be cured?*

A. Although there is no known cure for epilepsy, seizures in most people
can be partially or fully controlled with treatment.

*Q. Is epilepsy a lifelong condition?*

A. Not necessarily. Many people with epilepsy do not have seizures
throughout their entire lives.

*Q. Does a person with epilepsy have "fits"?*

A. A person with epilepsy experiences recurrent seizures; the outdated
term *fits* suggests a person is hysterical or has gone mad—which is
definitely not the case.

*Q. Will a person with epilepsy become mentally retarded?*

A. Epilepsy does not lead to mental retardation.

Q. *Is epilepsy a mental or emotional illness?*

A. No. It is a physical condition in which seizures are caused by excessive discharges of electricity in the brain.

Q. *Can a person die from epilepsy?*

A. Some people have seizures that are strong enough or prolonged enough to kill them. Others might have a fatal accident during a seizure, such as while climbing a high ladder or driving. But most people with epilepsy do not face life-threatening risks.

## Causes of Epilepsy and Seizures

There are many possible causes of epileptic seizures. Anything that leads to an abnormal pattern of neuron activity, such as a brain injury at birth, a head injury due to a car accident, or a brain tumor, can cause epilepsy. Genes can play a role, with some people inheriting a predisposition for a gene disorder that leads to abnormal brain activity.

## Read This!

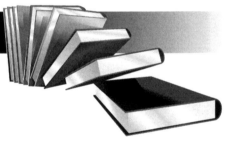

*This Ordinary Life* (Lumini Books, 2015), a novel by Jennifer Walkup, begins with the teenage narrator Jasmine Torres practicing early in the morning for an audition to win a scholarship for an internship at radio station WYN60 in New York City. The trip to the radio station is planned for that day. Jasmine has some broadcasting experience as morning host of Benton High School's radio show. Plus she is taking a high school class in radio broadcasting, and her dream is to be a topnotch DJ in New York City. Pursuing that dream is the basis of the story, but to make it happen she must overcome one obstacle after another.

The first chapter of the novel depicts Jasmine's "utterly craptastic" day. Before she leaves for school, Jennifer wakes her seven-year-old brother Danny, who has epilepsy. Jennifer makes sure he takes his meds, helps him get dressed, and fixes his breakfast and school lunch. Then she tries to rouse her alcoholic mother who is passed out on the couch, and reminds her to watch out for Danny. She rushes out the door to her boyfriend Sebastian's home to get a ride to school, only to find a shocking scene: he's in his bedroom engaged in sex with a girl whose "skinny fake-tan legs" protrude from the side of his bed. Then Jasmine's cell phone rings, and she learns that her brother has had a seizure and an ambulance is on the way.

As Jasmine tries to control her rage and disappointment over Sebastian, who is immediately an ex-boyfriend, she rushes back home and rides in the ambulance with her young brother to the hospital. While there, she observes another patient in the room with her brother—a cute teenage boy with bushy blonde hair. She learns later that his name is Wes, a funny, hang-loose guy, and that he, too, has epilepsy.

Part of the storyline in this novel is about the relationship between Jasmine and Wes. Jasmine is reluctant to even think about a new male friend, but as time goes by the two communicate via humorous text messages. Eventually, Jasmine accepts Wes as *just* a friend and insists that they should not have a real date.

Meantime, she attempts to keep focused on her dream, but she has missed out on the trip to New York because of Danny's seizure. She dearly loves and adores her little brother and would not think of leaving him in the care of her drunken mother. Jasmine is both mom and big sister to her little brother.

So much is on Jasmine's shoulders that she longs for an ordinary life. In spite of her problems, however, she still keeps hoping that her dream will come true. That hope is her strength and carries her forward. But revealing the ending would be a spoiler. Just read it!

---

Brain infections such as encephalitis and meningitis are responsible for some seizures, and people with AIDS, tuberculosis, or Jakob-Crutzfeldt disease may develop epilepsy. In the late stages of Alzheimer's, about one-third of those with this degenerative brain disease are likely to have seizures. Alcohol and other drug abuse can cause brain damage leading to epileptic seizures. A variety of other medical problems such as diabetes (high levels of glucose or sugar in the blood due to lack of insulin) or hypoglycemia (low blood sugar) can cause seizures, but not necessarily the chronic seizures of epilepsy. Once the medical problem is corrected, the seizures stop.

While neurologists, especially *epileptologists* who specialize in epilepsy, can pinpoint the cause for the disorder in some people, they are unable to determine what provokes epilepsy in a majority of the cases. The unknown factors leading to this brain disorder may contribute to the myths and prejudices surrounding epilepsy that persist to this day.

# WHAT HAPPENS?

*"Epilepsy has been very hard for me because for some reason,*
*I always thought of myself as broken, or weird, even alone. Then I learned that*
*1 in 26 people statistically will develop epilepsy in their life times."*
—Rachel, whose personal story is online[1]

Some people with epilepsy, whether school-age or adult, are unable to talk or write about their experiences with epileptic seizures. But others share what happened to them because they say it could help people struggling with their fears and negative feelings about epilepsy. Their stories also can have a widespread impact because they encourage donations and support for organizations and foundations seeking awareness and cures for epilepsy.

Those who share their experiences may not remember anything about the minutes or seconds before having a seizure. A seizure may happen when the person is asleep. Or there might be a sudden loss of consciousness. However, some people have *auras*, or unusual indicators before a seizure. These are described as a sour or bitter taste in the mouth, nausea, a "tight" feeling in the pit of the stomach, a tingling in the limbs, an intense ringing in the ears, or an unusual smell. Other common experiences just before a seizure include getting light-headed, breaking into a sweat, feeling extreme fear, getting depressed, struggling to talk, being unable to concentrate, and shaking.

On the website LivingWellwithEpilepsy.com, Emily wrote in 2016 about what happened to her before a seizure:

> I would get a feeling of fear; it was overwhelming and sometimes unbearable. I didn't want to leave the house. . . . I was crippled with Anxiety. Right before my seizure I would feel disconnected. It would feel as if I were watching my life from outside my body, and that I was not really there. At one point I could not even use the toilet because . . . it looked so big that I was afraid I would fall in and not be able to escape. I would often

repeatedly do something with no control, like clapping my hands together, wipe them down or make chewing motions.[2]

## First Aid or No Aid?

Not everyone who has a seizure needs first aid. Usually people who experience partial seizures and "blank out" only need emotional support and reassurance after they begin to respond to those around them. Sometimes helpers call 911 for an ambulance immediately, but experts say emergency service is not usually necessary—unless the seizure lasts more than five minutes or if the person has repeated seizures without regaining consciousness, is pregnant, or has signs of injury.

There are times when someone who witnesses a tonic-clonic seizure can be helpful. People having such a seizure may fall; they may begin to jerk uncontrollably, foam at the mouth, and cry out. A first-time observer of a convulsion may become frightened and try to provide aid. But there are dos and don'ts regarding assistance for an epileptic seizure.

First, an observer should never put an object in a seizing person's mouth. It's a common myth that during a convulsion a person will "swallow" his or her tongue. This is not only wrong, but it's dangerous to try to prevent it from happening—the tongue cannot be swallowed, and the person having a seizure is likely to suffer an injury to the mouth or break teeth from the clenched object. In addition, a helper is likely to be bitten!

Here's what experts say should and should not be done:

Do place a pillow or other cushion under the person's head.
Don't try to restrain a person; a seizure must end naturally.
Do loosen tight neckwear.
Don't leave a person alone; stay with him or her until the seizure ends.
Do clear the area of sharp objects.
Don't try to make the person drink anything.
Do look for an epilepsy medical identification tag.

When people have seizures and cannot respond, identification (ID) bracelets, necklaces, and anklets can alert helpers or medical professionals to their condition. Some IDs may be purple, the color symbolizing epilepsy. ID tags also may be personalized with information regarding a patient's primary doctor or specialist and the type of seizure disorder. For example, a tag might be engraved with "Mary Smith Epilepsy on Tegretol" along with a doctor's name and phone number. One source for epilepsy IDs and information about medical alerts is http://www.americanmedical-id.com/epilepsy.

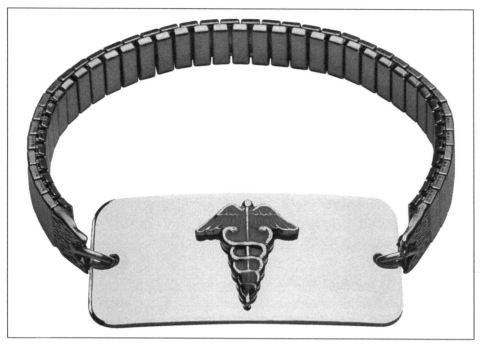

A person with epilepsy should wear an ID bracelet, necklace, or other tag so that helpers can be alerted to their condition.

## Canine Seizures

Yes, dogs have seizures similar to those that humans experience. A common epileptic condition in dogs is called *idiopathic epilepsy*, which is an inherited disorder in some breeds. Canine seizures can appear as dramatic and violent as human seizures. A legend, like the human myth, still prevails that when a dog has a seizure it will swallow its tongue. That falsehood prompts some people to try to put something in the dog's mouth, but veterinarian Ernest Ward wrote, "If you put your fingers or an object into its mouth, you will not help your pet and you run a high risk of being bitten very badly or of injuring your dog. The important thing is to keep the dog from falling or hurting itself by knocking objects onto itself. As long as it is on the floor or ground, there is little chance of harm occurring." If a dog has more than one seizure a month, a cluster of seizures, or a prolonged grand mal, veterinarians may prescribe anticonvulsant medications.[a]

# It Happened to Them

## *Sean*

Sean McGarrahan, a computer specialist who coauthored the original edition of this book, does not remember any warning before having his first seizure, which occurred about six months after his sixteenth birthday:

> The last thing I remember that Sunday morning was reading the Sunday comics. The next thing I know I'm in a daze. I can tell by the sound that the front door is open and that a vehicle with power generators—which I correctly assume to be an ambulance—is outside. But I still can't focus my thoughts. I know I'm on the floor, very weak and that I can't get up. Finally, I hear someone say, "OK, he's coming around now. What's his name? ('Sean') Sean, do you know what day it is?" "Saturday," I manage to mumble. "OK, one day off." I actually heard the paramedic say that. All this time, my mind is doing a continuous systems check. I can think, but I can't act.
>
> Gradually my mind started to clear. I recognized where I was and what was happening. Somewhere in this, they told me I had had a seizure. I just sort of accepted that, not really knowing the implications in my current state of mind.

After an overnight stay in the hospital, Sean was then referred to a pediatric neurologist. As he explained with a bit of irony,

> Pediatric neurologists handle patients up to age 17. I was 16 and a half. While I wasn't the oldest patient they had, I was considerably older than most of the other patients. Most of the chairs in the waiting area functioned better as footrests for me. And I found that reading literature in the waiting room was, oddly enough, medically oriented—written by some doctor named Seuss. I really couldn't understand why anyone would want to do a study on green eggs. Probably a federal grant.
>
> I was quite fortunate to be assigned to a neurologist, who was willing to talk frankly with me about my condition. He started me on the standard series of tests available at that time: blood work, computed tomography (CT) scan—a brain scan that shows the structure of the brain, and electroencephalograms (EEGs)—tests that record brain waves. We found that there actually was a brain inside my skull (a surprise to some); and that it did function, if not quite properly.

Sean's EEG showed an irregularity, but it wasn't conclusive. However, he soon learned that he suffered from tonic-clonic seizures. Nevertheless, as Sean put it, "they didn't know why I was having grand mal seizures." To this day, no one has been able to figure out why his seizures occurred, which is a complication, "but it doesn't make the disorder any more severe in reality," he said.[3]

When Sean first started having seizures, he took Depakote, a standard procedure for his type of epilepsy at the time, but he had another seizure.

My dosage was increased, but I still had another seizure. My doctor then switched me to Tegretol. That appeared to be working, but one day I noticed some spots on my arm. At my next appointment, I learned that I was allergic to Tegretol and was switched to Dilantin. I had a few more seizures after that, but once the dosage was increased, I stopped having seizures—for a while.

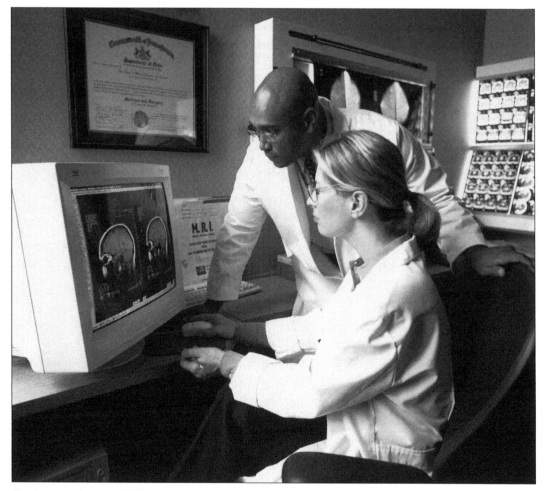

Doctors review an MRI scan.

Sean's medications were changed several times and gabapentin was added. But, he said, "My mind was really affected . . . so I stopped taking my medication altogether, without telling my doctor. NOT SMART—I DON'T RECOMMEND THIS" (Sean's emphasis). He eventually told his doctor and got back on track with his medications.[4]

## Barbara

In an article for Epilepsy.com, Barbara recalled her first seizure.

> I was officially diagnosed with epilepsy when I was 18, but, in hindsight, I realize I had my first seizures while I was still in high school. At 14, I remember standing in my bathroom admiring my cute new haircut, then coming to with a large lump on my forehead from blacking out and hitting my head on our porcelain sink. At 17, I remember standing in my bedroom getting ready for work and then lying on my bed looking up at my uncle, who had come to pick me up, and being unable to recognize him. I have no memory of what happened in between.

Barbara explained that she spent her teenage years staying close to home. But she went on to graduate from college, get married, and hold jobs. She wrote that she "had grand mal seizures in hotels, on an escalator, at two jobs (once in the middle of a presentation), in the airport, at my in-laws' house, at my house, at my mom's house, in the elevator at college, on a moving treadmill, and while I was pregnant. In other words, I lived life with epilepsy." Barbara emphasized that her story was just one of many, "but so many people fear their lives are over when they're diagnosed with epilepsy. I want them to know that doesn't have to be true."[5]

## Drake

Drake, a seventeen-year-old high school student, football player, and wrestler with a 3.453 grade point average, talked to a local Lake Station, Indiana, reporter in 2015 about his experiences with epilepsy. He explained what happened in 2011 while playing football: "I was getting ready to snap the ball and I kind of zoned out. . . . I went into my own world, and I never snapped the ball. I came out of this zone and everyone on the team was upset with me. I didn't know why they were upset. The coach took me out of the game. He talked to my parents and told them he thought I had a concussion."

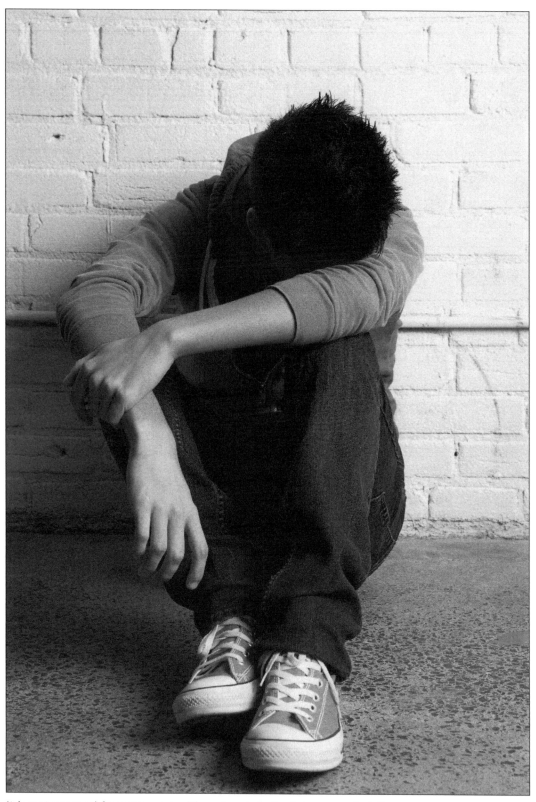

It is not unusual for someone with epilepsy to feel depressed at times.

After visits to the hospital and doctors and numerous tests, Drake learned that he had epilepsy. "I didn't even know what epilepsy was," he told the reporter. "I was scared. I went through a period of depression. I felt different from everyone else. I didn't even know anybody who had epilepsy. . . . I didn't know what it was going to mean for my life. I wondered if I would be able to play ball or hang out with my friends. I felt restricted from everything I wanted to do. I had to take pills every day; none of my friends had to do that."

With the help of medication, Drake snapped out of his depression, and he took a big step forward. "In March 2013, he went to the school board and told them about epilepsy and his desire to make more people aware of the [disorder]." Drake told the board that there probably were other teens who were depressed about having epilepsy and the school could have a "purple day"—the color for epilepsy—to raise awareness of epilepsy. He also spoke to the Indiana Senate about epilepsy and represented Indiana at the Epilepsy Foundation of America's Public Policy Institute/Teens Speak Up program.[6]

## Sophie

Sophie was seventeen years old in 2013 when she wrote about her experience on LivingWellwithEpilepsy.com. Originally from Maryland, Sophie moved to Geneva, Switzerland, when her father changed jobs. While she was in sixth grade, Sophie had a grand mal seizure in class and was diagnosed with epilepsy. "[My seizure] was a pretty scary time for everyone, especially my family. We had no way of predicting that I would have epilepsy. We had no family history of it." She added,

> Waking up in the hospital was shocking and really confusing to say the least. I knew what a seizure was but didn't understand why I had one. . . . When my neurologist told me I had epilepsy I was SO embarrassed. As if it wasn't bad enough having my entire class watch me shaking and convulsing passed out on the floor, now I had admit to having some . . . condition? Disease? . . . The doctors ran tests such as EEGs and MRIs to investigate what was wrong with my brain. . . . After even more tests, it was confirmed that the seizures were, in fact, coming from my temporal lobe. A year or so later, we would discover a cyst that existed around my left temporal lobe. . . . Four more grand mals and countless absence seizures later, I had brain surgery [in 2013]. The cyst in my brain was removed at the Cleveland Clinic in Ohio. . . .
>
> Although the odds are in my favor, I won't know whether or not I am completely seizure free for a while. Whether or not I am seizure free, I am

thankful every day for my amazing family and friends who love and support me through thick and thin.[7]

## *Layna*

When she was fourteen years old, Layna had her first seizure and then had another one at age fifteen, when she was diagnosed with epilepsy. She was told that her daily life would not be affected. But, as she wrote on CureEpilepsy.org, "Even though I could do a lot of the same things my life wasn't the same at all. I had to live in this world where I thought people would look at me like I was a freak because I had epilepsy. It was a daily struggle at first because I never was on medications before so I had to constantly be reminded that I needed to take my medicine." Layna described what happened to her in 2011 when she was eighteen. "I was straightening my hair with my flat iron and I had a seizure in the middle of it and fell on my flat iron and it burned the side of my face. I was so out of it I did not even know when I finally came back to my senses."

Her mother and stepfather took her to the hospital where she was treated for "a third degree burn and the burn killed all the nerves in that area of my face and I had to have surgery. . . . Because of that burn I missed the last two weeks of my senior year because I was in and out of the hospital, doctors' offices, and my neurologist's office." In spite of the trauma and disappointments, Layna graduated from high school and went on to college. She urges people to "support epilepsy and help find a cure."[8]

## Teen Support Groups

Adolescents and young adults with epilepsy who find it difficult to openly discuss their disorder often can find help through support groups. Some support groups can be accessed on the Internet where chat rooms offer people with epilepsy an opportunity to ask questions, share information, and "talk" informally with one another. Other support groups form so that people can meet face-to-face and share their concerns.

Numerous support groups that cater to teens with epilepsy have formed across the United States and in other countries. Such groups are initiated by affiliates of the Epilepsy Foundation, hospitals, or religious organizations, or by individual teens. Most teen support groups include no more than a dozen young people with a facilitator, or group leader. The facilitator is usually a health care professional, social worker, or other person knowledgeable about epilepsy and the psychological

## Read It!

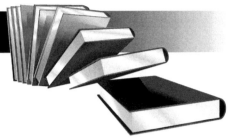

In times past, writers such as William Shake-speare, Fyodor Dostoyevsky, and Charles Dickens created characters who had epilepsy. Such characters also appear in some modern-day novels such as *100 Sideways Miles* described in chapter 5. Another example is *Takedown* (Banks Channel Books, 1999) by E. M. J. Benjamin, a pen name for a two-person writing team, one of them a high school wrestling coach.

In the story, seventeen-year-old Jake is the central character, a high school wrestler whose coach constantly drills the team on takedowns, the moment when a wrestler takes his opponent to the mat. Jake may complain about practice, but he's dedicated to winning the high school wrestling title.

After several seizures, which are preceded by auras, a "rotten-cheese smell," as Jake describes it, he learns he has epilepsy. His reaction mirrors many real-life cases of young people who receive this diagnosis. Members of Jake's family—Chopper, a younger brother, and his parents—also react in a typical fashion. However, Chopper, a computer whiz, has searched the Internet for information on seizures, sharing his knowledge with Jake, who doesn't really want to believe what his brother tells him.

The story realistically portrays Jake's attempts to deal with epilepsy. At first he is in denial; then he's angry and asks the "Why me?" question in a variety of different ways. Jake decides not to tell anyone he has epilepsy—not his friends, not his coach. He calls himself "The Great Liar" and uses numerous subterfuges to keep from revealing his disorder. Jake also has to deal with taking his medication daily and, as happens in real life, he sometimes forgets, triggering a seizure one evening while out of town for a wrestling meet.

Jake can no longer hide his condition, so he withdraws. His coach, friends, and father try to bring Jake back. Eventually he does stop feeling sorry for himself. He comes to terms with epilepsy and gains control of his life.

and social concerns facing teens with epilepsy. Such a person is able to correct erroneous information about epilepsy and lead group discussions.

Topics frequently discussed are overprotective parents, employment, sexuality, dating, driving, and explaining seizures to classmates, teachers, coworkers, and others. Within a support group, young people can learn to speak freely and develop social skills and self-confidence. Teens in support groups also learn how to deal with others' prejudices about epilepsy and how to counteract misconceptions with facts.

# DIAGNOSING AND TREATING EPILEPSY

*"Having epilepsy has . . . shaped why I want to become a nurse.
I want to help others who have an illness. In my personal experience,
when I visited doctors when I was younger, I felt that sometimes I was
treated as a 'medical case' versus a person living with epilepsy."*
—Monique, a twenty-two-year-old college student[1]

Treatment for a person who has had a seizure begins with determining whether the seizure is actually due to epilepsy. One of the first tools in diagnosing epilepsy is collecting accurate information about what a patient felt and was doing before and after losing consciousness. Obviously someone who is unconscious cannot provide any of the details, but an eyewitness may be able to give a doctor important information.

That eyewitness for a young child is likely to be a parent. Chandler Jahnke's mother, for example, vividly recalls what happened in 2010 when her ten-year-old daughter had her first seizure. "All of a sudden, she collapsed on the floor," Jackie recalled, "and we didn't know what was going on. It was terrifying." For more than two years, "Chandler and her family struggled with her neurologists to find a medication that would control her seizures and not have debilitating side effects. . . . After two and a half years they finally found what they were looking for," according to EpilepsyChicago.org.[2] As a teenager, Chandler became an activist for the Epilepsy Foundation, and in 2015, she attended the Teens Speak Up Conference in Washington, DC.

## Questions Doctors Ask

When a parent consults a physician about treatment for a child with seizures, the doctor will likely ask questions like these:

When did the event (seizure) take place?
Were there any warning signs that the child was losing consciousness?
How long was she or he unconscious?
How did the child or teenager act during and after the seizure?
Do other family members have epilepsy?
Were there any problems at birth?

While questioning a teenager or adult, a doctor will ask the patient questions, such as: Do you use drugs or have a history of alcohol abuse? Have you had any head injuries? Have you had meningitis? After clinical information is gathered, a doctor may order a thorough neurological examination, which commonly includes an electroencephalogram (EEG).

## About the EEG

The EEG is a valuable and painless test in diagnosing epilepsy. It can be administered while the patient is awake or asleep. The normal waking EEG detects and records the brain's electrical patterns—brain waves. Gel is applied to about two dozen small disks called electrodes that are attached to various locations on the scalp. The gel does not damage the hair—it can be washed out. Wires from the disks are connected to an EEG machine, which records the brain's electrical patterns and stores them on a computer or prints out the brain waves on paper.

As electrodes pick up the tiny electrical charges in the brain, the EEG amplifies these charges, sending them to a series of pens that track the electrical activity that appears as a graph on a computer screen, or as a recording that may be printed out on paper. A patient has to lie quietly during an EEG test, because body movements could alter the results. But the technician administering the test asks a patient to perform several actions that can stimulate brain waves, such as breathing rapidly, opening and closing the eyes, and looking at flashing lights. A neurologist who analyzes an EEG will distinguish between what is normal and abnormal in a person's brain waves.

However, an EEG is not flawless; it may not show an abnormal pattern even though a person has epilepsy. When there is uncertainty about a patient's condition, a doctor may have a patient wear or carry a portable EEG device to record brain waves over a twenty-four- or forty-eight-hour period. Video monitoring along with an EEG test during a seizure might also be ordered. In some cases, this requires that a person be deprived of sleep, which could initiate a seizure; a video camera then records a patient's activity during an EEG.

A patient may have to go to an Epilepsy Monitoring Unit (EMU) in the hospital for another type of video monitoring. The stay in an EMU ranges from several days to two weeks. During this time, physicians may instruct patients taking antiseizure drugs to decrease their dosages or discontinue their medications so that seizures can occur. Because patients are constantly wired to video and EEG monitoring equipment, they are not able to move around much, spending most of the time sitting in a bed or a chair. Electrodes stay on the head during the entire monitoring period, so patients can't wash their hair or take showers.

## Other Diagnostic Tools

Along with EEGs, other important tools in diagnosing epilepsy are brain scans. The most frequently used scans include computed tomography (CT) and magnetic resonance imaging (MRI). CT and MRI scans show the brain's structure, helping a doctor identify abnormalities such as cysts and tumors. CT scans use X-rays; MRI scans do not.

MRI scans produce more detailed images of the brain. If a teenager (or any other patient) is having one of these tests, she or he lies on a scanning table that slides into a tunnel-like machine. When an MRI scan is performed, a magnetic field is created and radio waves are beamed at the brain. Small particles called protons within the brain's atoms produce radio waves that are picked up and measured by a sensitive device and then analyzed by a computer that creates detailed pictures of the brain. In people with epilepsy, an MRI can show a scar, lesion, or other structural cause for seizures. "However, many people have brain lesions without having epilepsy, and many people with epilepsy do not have any scars or lesions on their brain," according to the UK's Epilepsy Society.[3]

## Common Treatments

If a person is diagnosed with epilepsy, the most common treatment is daily use of anticonvulsant drugs. The first antiepileptic drugs were bromides, introduced in 1857 by Sir Charles Locock, an English physician. Locock found that sodium bromide, a sedative, reduced epileptic seizures. Other medications introduced in the early 1900s were phenobarbital and phenytoin, known by the trade name Dilantin.

Currently drugs have both trade names, which are capitalized, and generic names. They include Felbatol (felbamate), Neurontin (gabapentin), Lamictal (lamotrigine), Topamax (topiramate), Gabitril (tiagabine), Tegretol (carbamazepine), Depakote (divalproex sodium), Keppra (levetiracetam), and Zonagran (zonisamide). As of 2016, there were at least twenty different antiseizure drugs.

How does a doctor determine which medication to prescribe? It depends on the kind of seizure a person is having. Different drugs are designed to control different types of seizures. Some of these medications can have unpleasant to debilitating side effects, such as migraine headaches, suicidal thoughts, jaundice, blurred vision, dizziness, rashes, liver toxicity, insomnia, confusion, and difficulty concentrating. Many doctors believe that the side effects are acceptable if there is an overall reduction of seizures.

Diverse people require different dosages of medications. Because of the way people's bodies metabolize or process medicine, the resulting amount (or level) left in the bloodstream can vary. Some people can take a low dose and get a therapeutic level; others may need a higher dose of medication. People with epilepsy may have to adjust their medications often in order to control their seizures. Or a doctor may prescribe a combination of drugs.

## Medical Cannabis

Treating epilepsy with cannabis or marijuana (they have the same meaning) has long been controversial. Using this weed, which grows wild and also is cultivated, for any purpose has been federally banned since 1970 with passage of the Controlled Substances Act. The law regulates the manufacture and distribution of drugs like sedatives, depressants, and stimulants. It classifies drugs into five

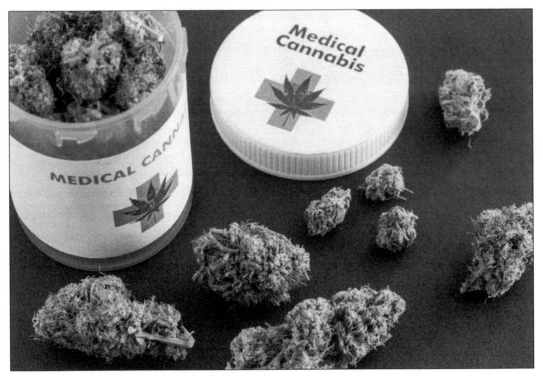

It has become more common for doctors to prescribe cannabis for a variety of medical issues, including epilepsy. ©iStock.com/tvirbickis

different schedules based on their potential for abuse. Marijuana is classified as Schedule I—that is, a substance or chemical "with no currently accepted medical use and a high potential for abuse," according to the U.S. Drug Enforcement Administration.

However, in December 2015, the U.S. Congress renewed an amendment to the Commerce, Justice and Science (CJS) Appropriations bill. The bipartisan amendment prohibits the U.S. Justice Department, including the Drug Enforcement Administration, from interfering with *state* medical marijuana laws. The legislation prohibits the federal government from using any funds to arrest or prosecute medical marijuana patients or providers that are in compliance with their state laws. But marijuana is still listed as a Schedule I drug. Unless marijuana is deleted from Schedule I classification, there is still a question about whether cannabis users, providers, and growers can be prosecuted by federal authorities.

## Cannabidiol (CBD)

Cannabis is a plant that grows in almost any non-extreme climate and environment, and contains numerous chemical compounds, one of which is delta-9-tetrahydrocannabinol (THC), known for producing a variety of sensory and psychological effects—in other words, a "high." Cannabis also contains cannabidiol (CBD), which calms the nervous system. CBD oil is extracted from the plant and can provide relief for countless people who suffer from a great variety of health problems, including arthritis, cancer, epilepsy, and sleep disorders.

Lora and Roger Barbour of New Jersey, began administering cannabis oil to their teenage daughter Genny, who is autistic and epileptic. She has had multiple seizures each day, but with the marijuana treatment of four doses each day, Genny had fewer seizures. Her mother said Genny actually went eight days without an attack. But Larc School for disabled children in Bellmawr, which Genny attends, would not allow her to take her needed dose at noon. As a result, "There were horrible behaviors in the afternoon and more seizures," her father told a *Courier-Post* reporter. "They were locking her in a restraint chair. She was throwing tantrums, biting herself, giving herself bruises. . . . The doctor, along with us, came to the conclusion that it (medical marijuana) was wearing off."[4] So Roger Barbour, an attorney, went to court three times in an attempt to allow Genny's mother or a school nurse to administer the cannabis oil at the school.

In Barbour's latest lawsuit in June 2015, a state judge ruled that state and federal laws forbid the use of medical marijuana on school grounds. In order for Genny to get her noon dose, her mother picked her up at school and took her home for the treatment. "The family's plight and the publicity surrounding it prompted the state legislature to pass a bill . . . that would require schools to establish rules allowing students with developmental disabilities to consume edible cannabis on campus," according to the news report.[5] In November 2015, New Jersey governor Chris Christie signed a law that "requires all school districts in New Jersey to adopt rules that permit children with developmental disabilities to consume cannabis oil or another edible cannabis product."[6]

## Charlotte's Web

Dr. Sanjay Gupta, a neurologist and chief medical correspondent for CNN, has produced three documentaries that include coverage of medical marijuana use—*Weed*, *Weed 2*, and *Weed 3*. In the films and in statements on CNN, Gupta recalled that he had once been against medical cannabis but had a "turn around" in 2013. "At the time it was a lonely place to hold a supportive position on medical marijuana. Hardly any government officials would agree to sit down and be interviewed on the topic. Even patients I spoke to were reluctant to share their stories," he said. But then he met and observed Charlotte Figi, who after taking cannabidiol went from having three hundred seizures a week to just one or two a month.[7]

Charlotte, the daughter of Matt and Paige Figi of Colorado, was born in 2006 and at only a few months old began having seizures. She was hospitalized numerous times and given many different medications for epilepsy, some of them strong barbiturates. A special diet helped for a time, but the seizures returned and were constant. There seemed to be no treatment options, and Charlotte began to decline mentally and physically. But the Figis continued to look for help, eventually finding a doctor to prescribe cannabis oil, which they purchased from a legal dispensary in Colorado. To everyone's amazement the seizures stopped.

However, the Figis' supply of oil ran out—until they heard about the five Stanley brothers who "were crossbreeding a strain of marijuana . . . high in CBD and low in THC." But the brothers didn't know what to do with it. "No one wanted it; [we] couldn't sell it," one of the brothers told Saundra Young of CNN. So the Stanley brothers founded Realm of Caring Foundation that provides cannabis to adults and children suffering from a host of diseases, including epilepsy. The marijuana strain was named Charlotte's Web "after the little girl who is getting her life back one day at a time."[8] Dr. Gupta is now an outspoken advocate for legalizing medical marijuana.

Congressional members have also added their voices. Senators Cory Booker, Kirsten Gillibrand, and Rand Paul introduced a bill in 2015 titled the Compassionate Access, Research Expansion and Respect States (CARERS) Act. If passed, the legislation would "end federal prohibition of medical marijuana and

## A Federal Cannabis Farm

A federal cannabis farm is located at the University of Mississippi in Oxford, and is part of the school's research lab. It is the only facility allowed to grow cannabis under the Controlled Substances Act. Officially known as the Marijuana Research Project, it began in 1968. The project is overseen by the National Institutes on Drug Abuse. "Between its inception and 2007, the farm supported only a small amount of research because there was little to no demand by scientists," CNN reported. "In Spring 2013, when Dr. Sanjay Gupta first visited the Marijuana Project, there was nothing growing in the fields because of this lack of demand. But when he returned a year and a half later, it was a much different story. Acres of the farm were teeming with research-grade medical cannabis in anticipation of a renewed interest in government-approved research."[a]

In 2015, the University of Mississippi received $68.8 million from the federal government to grow marijuana and analyze it.[b]

also introduce a host of other reforms aiming to curb restrictions on its transport, prescription and availability," according to MSNBC.[9]

As of June 2016, a total of twenty-five states and the District of Columbia had legalized the purchase and use of medical marijuana. Ohio was the most recent state to pass such a law, which Governor John Kasich signed in May 2016. Individual states that have legalized medical marijuana are Alaska, Arizona, California, Colorado, Connecticut, Delaware, Hawaii, Illinois, Maine, Maryland, Massachusetts, Michigan, Minnesota, Montana, Nevada, New Hampshire, New Jersey, New Mexico, New York, Ohio, Oregon, Pennsylvania, Rhode Island, Vermont, and Washington. The amounts that consumers are allowed are posted online. For example, Colorado allows a person to legally possess two ounces of usable marijuana and six plants. Consumers in Massachusetts can have a sixty-day supply for personal medical use. In Washington State, an individual consumer can purchase twenty-four ounces of usable marijuana and fifteen plants.[10]

## Keeping a Diary or Log

To help in epilepsy treatment, a diary or log can be beneficial for both the patient and his or her doctor. Here is a *fictitious* example. It notes the length of the episode, the date and time, a description of the seizure, recovery time, and circumstances of the day. Medications and their level should be included, but those vary by individual so are not suggested in this example.

Apr 19, 3:00 p.m.—in college game room, playing pinball, alone. Sz. Awoke soon after. Hit head hard, but no sign of concussion. Phenobarbital level measured, barely therapeutic. Had not missed dosage. Dr. @ ER directed change to higher dosage.

Apr 25, 7:00 p.m.—at video store. Sz outside on sidewalk. Chipped/cracked tooth, bloody nose. Recovered fairly quickly. Waiting for ER Dr.

May 10, 1:00 p.m.—at beach house. Had not missed medication. Was sleeping, wakened by phone, noted usual effects. Did not go to hosp.

Nov 7, 3:00 p.m.—in computer room, while home sick. Fell forward, hit face and chest on computer desk. Not feeling well for several days before.

Nov 14, 7:00 a.m.—at home in bed, sleeping, after being up late. Recovery slow. 17 min. before lucid. Had taken medication prior. Upset stomach, no supper previous evening. Had taken normal doses previous morning and noontime.

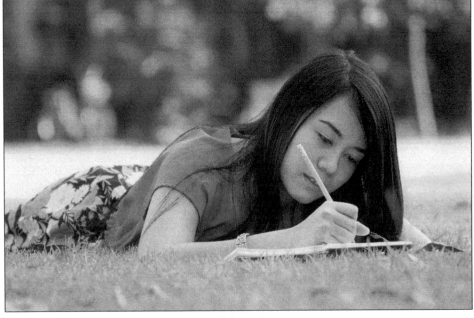

Keeping a journal about your seizures can help your doctor determine the proper course of treatment. ©iStock.com/Meal_MeaW

## The Ketogenic Diet

A treatment for some young people with a severe form of epilepsy, especially those with intractable epilepsy, is the ketogenic diet, which in some forms has been used since biblical times. The modern ketogenic diet was introduced in the 1920s before antiseizure medications were widely available. It is high in fats (such as vegetable oils and cream) and low in carbohydrates and protein. Carbohydrates are made up of sugars (glucose), and if they are decreased in the diet and fat is substituted instead, the body has no glucose source. For survival, the body breaks down fats instead of carbohydrates for fuel, producing a condition in the body known as ketosis.

There are numerous drawbacks to this diet, however. First and foremost, it is difficult to maintain and requires eating a limited number of fatty foods. Food and liquid intake must be carefully calculated and monitored each day. Even the amount of sugar in a pill must be counted. Side effects from the diet can include nausea, stomach cramps, and nutritional deficiencies that inhibit growth. The diet should not be attempted without the guidance of health care professionals.

The British Epilepsy Society has a seizure diary on its website. The diary is in pdf format and pages can be printed out as needed. It includes detailed explanations on how to complete the various sections. In addition, there is an app that can be downloaded free on a smartphone.[11]

A U.S. version of a seizure diary appears on the Epilepsy Foundation's website. It is called "Epilepsy Foundation My Seizure Diary." To access the diary, individuals register, log in, and keep a record on a computer or (with an app) on a smartphone.[12]

# BRAIN SURGERY

·····································································

*"I've been riding the motorcycle a lot. . . . Looking forward to actually joining*
*the Marine Corps now that I'm able to, hanging out with friends,*
*going out and doing a lot of things I couldn't do before."*
—*eighteen-year-old Collin May after epileptic brain surgery*[1]

In some epilepsy cases, medication does little to control seizures, and brain surgery may be considered. Any surgery carries risks, and certainly brain surgery is a major undertaking. But the decision to treat epilepsy with surgery is only made after a detailed assessment of a patient. This involves a team of neurologists, neurosurgeons, social workers, and perhaps psychiatrists. These specialists carefully evaluate such factors as the frequency and severity of seizures, the risk of brain damage from frequent seizures, and what economic and social impact surgery would have on a person's family and quality of life.

As doctors for the Epilepsy Foundation put it, "Epilepsy treatment must consider a person's quality of life, not just the number of seizures. Both continued seizures and high doses of medication impose costs on all areas of a person's life—intellectual, psychological, social, educational, and employment." If surgery is an option, "studies have shown that the earlier surgery is performed, the better the outcome."[2]

WebMD reports that

the effectiveness of surgery varies, depending on the type of surgery, with success rates varying between 50% and 80%. Some people are completely free of seizures after surgery. For others, the frequency of seizures is significantly reduced. In some cases, surgery may not be successful and a second surgery (re-operation) may be recommended. Most patients will need to continue taking anti-seizure medication for a year or more after surgery. Once seizure control is established, medications may be reduced or eliminated.[3]

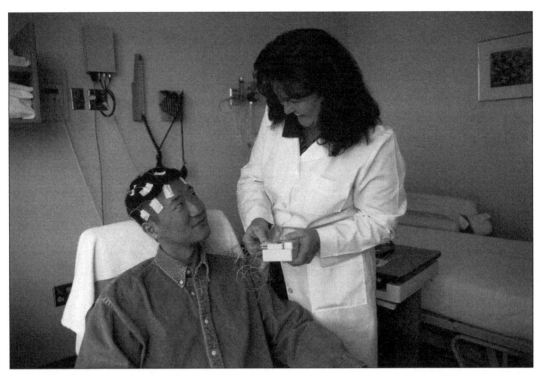

A doctor monitors epilepsy with EEG.

Patients who are candidates for brain surgery undergo numerous tests and are monitored intensively. The first test would likely be an EEG (electroencephalogram). An MRI would be performed to determine whether there are abnormalities such as tumors or scars that can prompt seizures. To locate the exact focus of seizures, doctors might implant electrodes into the brain or lay them on the surface of the brain to record brain activity, providing more information than is possible to obtain with an EEG. A test might be given in which the drug amobarbital is injected to locate areas of the brain controlling memory and speech. Surgeons would need such information to avoid operating on that part of the brain.

Psychiatric testing may also be done for some patients. A psychiatric assessment helps rule out a mental illness, such as severe depression, that would prevent surgery until the illness could be successfully treated. It would also determine whether a patient would follow the pre- and post-surgery procedures.

## Successful Brain Surgeries

Among successful surgeries to control seizures was one performed in late December 2015 for a Logansport, Louisiana, teenager named LaCameron Grant. He had been having seizures for five years and had been taking three antiseizure medications. But he continued to have unpredictable seizures—he had no auras or warnings that a seizure was about to happen.

He told reporter Segann March of the *Shreveport Times* that when he had seizures in public, people around him did not know what to do. "I kept wondering why people were so scared every time they thought I'd end up having a seizure. . . . They would just bug out, it was unfamiliar for them," he said.[4] Because of his seizures, LaCameron could not swim, play contact sports, or go to strobe light parties. Activities like these often spark seizures in some people with epilepsy.

After months of planning with a medical team, LaCameron underwent surgery. During a seven-hour operation, doctors used a computer-guided system to locate a tumor deep in the right side of the teenager's brain. Surgeons were able to remove the lesion, and LaCameron was able to go home a few days later. He told reporter Nick Lawton: "I feel very good. . . . I doubt most people would be just up and running four days after brain surgery!" Doctors planned to monitor LaCameron to make sure he continues to be seizure-free.[5]

Manhattan Beach, California, teenager Cailin Stroyke also had brain surgery to stop her seizures. She was having numerous events each day. Medication did not help and "doctors determined that her right temporal lobe was damaged when she was an infant, and her left temporal lobe had taken over its functions—mostly memory—at a young age," the *Daily Breeze* reported. Surgeons determined the location of the structural damage in Cailin's brain. And in May 2013, surgeons at the Ronald Reagan UCLA Medical Center removed one-eighth of her brain. She has been seizure-free ever since, and said, "Now a lot of my free time is spent doing charity work for the [Epilepsy] foundation. . . . I'd just like to give back. It sounds so cliché, but I know I am one of the luckier people. . . . I still have epilepsy, but there are kids who have it way worse who can't be operated on or the medications don't work, so they are living with having seizures every day."[6]

Another California teen who had surgery was Angel Ojeda of Los Altos. Angel's mother reported that her son "had intractable complex partial seizures. He had seizures on a weekly basis, sometimes clusters of up to ten in a day. He could not get through a full week of school without seizures, and often had seizures in front of his classmates. . . . He had weekly ambulance rides from school and he spent countless days in the hospital." In 2015, Angel had successful surgery at UC Irvine Medical Center. Since the surgery, he has been able to attend school on a regular basis and participate in track. He is also free of side effects of antiseizure medications as well as depression that often affects people with epilepsy.[7]

One more success story focused on eighteen-year-old Collin May of Ohio. He underwent laser surgery in 2016 at the Cleveland Clinic's Epilepsy Center. A news release from the clinic noted that May sometimes endured more than fifty seizures a day. "At night I would have the seizures and wouldn't get a lot of sleep at all and then I'd wake up and be tired and that would give me more seizures.

. . . And I would go to school and you know, getting a lecture in class, and I'd have another seizure," May said.[8]

During May's operation, doctors pinpointed the exact spot in the brain that was causing the seizures. Then the neurosurgeon inserted a tiny laser probe and heated the tissue around the probe, creating a small lesion. "Once doctors felt the area causing the seizures was completely burned away, they removed the probe and closed the incision with one stitch. . . . May hasn't had a seizure since his surgery," according to the news release.[9]

## It Happened to Billy

In February 2016, the British *Daily Mail* described how surgeons at Bristol Royal Hospital for Children used a robot in pioneering surgery. The surgical procedure was done to cure epileptic seizures that fifteen-year-old Billy Whitaker had been experiencing for eight years. Called robotic stereotactic EEG, a robot located the exact spot triggering Billy's seizures. According to the newspaper story, Billy was put under general anesthetic and doctors performed "a number of scans to create a 3D map of Billy's brain to identify the areas for 'interrogation', on January 14," adding,

> They then screwed a frame into his head using four pencil-lead thick screws to guide the robot to position the drill.
>
> The robot then provided a 3D trajectory of the place it was going to place the electrode, and positioned the 1mm [1/32 inch] thick drill bit ready for the surgeon.
>
> The high-tech machine drilled through the skin and skull, and then 3cm [1.18 inches] into the brain tissue in four difference locations, before then guiding in a silicon electrode.
>
> When Billy came round following the five-hour operation his epilepsy medication was reduced to bring on seizures—and he had nine attacks over three days.
>
> The electrodes—which were screwed onto his scalp—picked up the signals via the sensors along their length, pinpointing the exact location in his brain causing the attacks.

A week later, Billy went back under the knife where surgeons cut a "trap door" in his skull and cut out the finger-tip sized bit of brain which was causing his fits. [Note: the outdated term *fits* means seizures.]

On January 21, 2016, Billy told *Daily Mail* reporter Anne Hodgekiss, "Being seizure free means I will be able to take part in sports like football and rugby again. . . . It is exciting to be the first patient to have been treated at the hospital with this technique. . . . Although it is sometimes boring being monitored, the care I have received and the nurses who have treated me, have inspired me to look at the potential of working . . . in a hospital."[a]

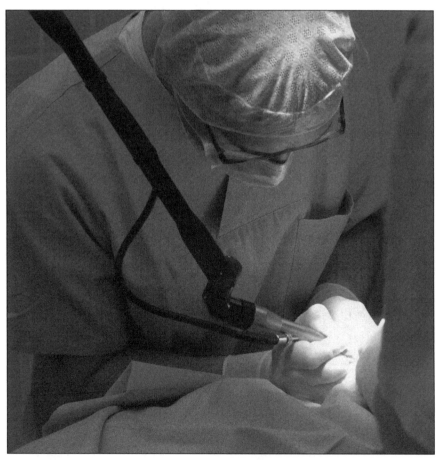

Doctors perform laser surgery to help control epileptic seizures. ©iStock .com/Falk Keinas

## Vagus Nerve Stimulation

Some people with medication-resistant forms of epilepsy are not eligible for brain surgery to eliminate seizures. In such cases, vagus nerve stimulation (VNS) may be a therapeutic strategy. The word *vagus* is Latin for wandering or straying. "There's one vagus nerve on each side of your body, running from your brain stem through your neck to your chest and abdomen," explains the Mayo Clinic.[10]

*Science News* describes the vagus nerve this way: "With outposts in nearly every organ and a direct line into the brain stem, the vagus nerve is the nervous system's superhighway. About 80 percent of its nerve fibers—or four of its five 'lanes'—drive information from the body to the brain. Its fifth lane runs in the opposite direction, shuttling signals from the brain throughout the body."[11]

People whose seizures are not helped by medication may have a VNS device surgically implanted under the skin of the chest (rather like a pacemaker). It is attached to the vagus nerve in the lower neck. The device delivers short bursts of electrical energy to the brain via the vagus nerve. On average, this stimulation reduces seizures by about 20 to 40 percent. Individuals usually cannot stop taking epilepsy medication because of the stimulator, but they often experience fewer seizures and they may be able to reduce the dosage of their medication.

## Read This!

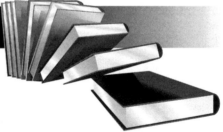

In the young adult novel *100 Sideways Miles* by Andrew Smith (Simon & Schuster, 2014), the story is told by teenager Finn Easton, who lives in Southern California. When he was only seven years old, Finn was injured while walking with his mother under a bridge. He was slammed to the ground by a dead horse that fell off a knackery truck hauling dead animals to a rendering plant. Finn's mother died from the impact of the horse. As a result of his injury, Finn developed epilepsy. He has pins in his back from surgery and a scar that looks like "colon, vertical slash, colon," or :|: that he calls "puncture-ation marks."[b] The marks are an integral part of the story.

Finn's father marries a nurse who cared for Finn during his long stay in the hospital, and both father and stepmother are vigilant about their teenage son's well-being, worrying about his seizures. In the story, Finn describes how his seizures come on. "I am just standing there, and first I smell something sweet—like flowers or maple syrup. Then I realize that I don't know the names for anything I am looking at. . . . Sounds, colors, textures, all mash together in an enormous symphonic assault on my senses as I shrink down smaller and smaller."[c] In some instances in the story, Finn's seizures happen at crucial and embarrassing times. But there is no mention of treatment, and his parents don't seem concerned about Finn's best friend, Cade Hernandez.

Cade is a beer drinker and raucous, uninhibited teenager, staging numerous stunts and bellowing obnoxious comments to anyone he dislikes. Hernandez is obsessed with erections and masturbation. Still, Cade is tolerated by the Eastons because Cade has a car and drives Finn to school (Finn cannot legally drive because of his seizures). Cade is the direct opposite of introverted Finn, who is cerebral and an avid reader. He has never had a girlfriend, until he meets and falls in love with Julia Bishop, who arrives in their California town from Chicago.

The novel is like a book within a book. Finn's father is an author who writes science fiction novels, one of which is the best-selling *The Lazarus Door* about aliens with wings who eat humans. The aliens are eventually destroyed, but one survives. He is named Finn and has epilepsy and wants to find his way out the Lazarus door.

The Finn Easton of *100 Sideways Miles* is convinced that his father has written about him and that he is a captive inside his father's novel. Indeed, *Lazarus Door* reflects the father's need to keep his son close so that he won't lose him as he lost his wife.

Nevertheless, Finn and Cade have numerous adventures, during which Finn counts off his time in miles. Early in the story, he reasons, "Distance is more important than time. Earth travels about twenty miles per second." So he figures "$\pi$, our distance from the sun, three hundred sixty-five days, and there you go." Thus his time is equated to "twenty miles, twenty miles" etc. [d] During the story, the miles (minutes, hours, days) pass and Finn escapes his father's book; he becomes his own person.

## Neurostimulation

Another surgically implanted device called a Neurostimulator analyzes brain activity patterns to detect a forthcoming seizure. The University of California, San Francisco (UCSF), is one of the few centers in the United States to provide a device called a NeuroPace Responsive Neurostimulation. It was approved by the U.S. Food and Drug Administration in late 2013.

The battery-driven device is implanted in the skull. "Wires or leads are connected to the Neurostimulator that is placed on the surface and/or inside the brain. The Neurostimulator monitors the electrical activity of the brain and detects abnormal activity that could lead to a seizure. When abnormal activity is detected, the Neurostimulator delivers electrical stimulation to the brain through the leads to prevent seizures," according to UCSF.[12]

# LIVING WITH EPILEPSY

*"To live in fear of Epilepsy is to live in fear of yourself."*
—*Gillian Mangan, University of Florida student*[1]

Most teenagers with epilepsy often feel helpless and frightened after they have seizures. They may be afraid to go out on their own. They may worry that they will forget their antiseizure medications. Many teens and adults with epilepsy fear they will have a seizure in public and that they will be embarrassed by their behavior.

Nineteen-year-old university student Samantha, who has epilepsy, wrote on the website CureEpilepsy.org:

When I have [a seizure], I feel helpless and scared, scared that I may not come out of the next one, or that I will have one in a place or situation that will potentially place me at risk, or my loved ones at risk of watching me and not being able to do anything. I have to admit, it is also humiliating . . . to be in that position, having crowds surround you and people who all of a sudden act very differently because of "this side of you" they have seen. It can be so confronting to see a grand mal/tonic clonic seizure, to watch someone you love convulse, eyes in the back of their head, foaming at the mouth, knowing you can do nothing. I have seen a video of myself having one, and I was vacant—just not there. It was a terribly scary thing to see.[2]

When families and friends of people witness a seizure, they may feel "edgy," not knowing what to expect or look for in regard to someone who has seizures. Frequently parents say they have difficulty accepting an epilepsy diagnosis. In some cases they don't really want to believe the doctors and are in denial at first. They may seek out support groups to help them deal with the reality. Parents also may feel guilty and believe they are responsible for a child's epilepsy. Or they raise their children to believe they are unable to accomplish much; as a result, by the time they are teenagers these young people have low opinions of themselves and may be very dependent on others.

## Accepting Lifestyle Changes

The teenage years are a time for many to rebel and to assert their individuality. It is not unusual for any young person (or adult, for that matter) with epilepsy to resent necessary adjustment to his or her daily routine. But refusing to accept lifestyle changes can have some dangerous consequences. For example, some teens try to assert their independence by not taking medication. But that can lead to a seizure. Drinking alcohol can also be a problem. Even if state laws permit teenage drinking, alcohol interacts with prescription drugs and could cause a seizure. On the positive side, getting plenty of sleep, eating nutritious food, following up with medical appointments, and joining support groups can help make life easier for someone with epilepsy.

On the other hand, some teenagers may have very supportive parents. Such parents are likely to avoid doing anything that would increase anxiety and do not discourage activities such as team sports unless doctors advise otherwise.

When people with epilepsy live alone, they usually have to make safety adjustments, such as not smoking or using matches, which can cause fires or burns during a seizure. Cooking also can be hazardous. One way to avoid spilling hot foods or boiling liquids is to place pots and pans on the back burner of a stove with the handles facing inward. An electric stove is preferable to a gas stove with flames. Using a microwave for cooking is even better.

An alarm or other device can be a reminder about bedtime, especially for people whose seizures are triggered by being overly tired. It is also important to avoid working on ladders or unprotected heights when alone. Another safety tip at home or work is to pad sharp corners, use nonslip carpets, and avoid scatter rugs.

## Embracing a "New Normal"

Gillian Mangan of Ocala, Florida, started a blog and a project that includes photographs of young people with epilepsy. She explained that the project was "constructed to highlight people with seizures who adjust their daily routine to the 'new normal' and are successful in their own way. The success may be minor

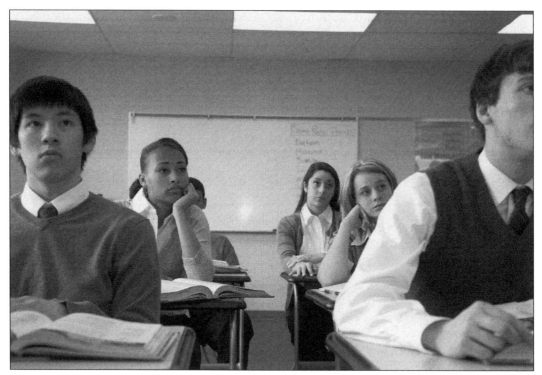

In most classrooms, a person with epilepsy is not easily identified, and some young people with epilepsy outgrow the disorder.

or it may be accomplishments made in their career, the key is to break the seizure stigma."[3]

On November 20, 2015, she wrote, "I have experienced four grand-mal seizures in a matter of six weeks. The last seizure occurred last night, leaving behind bruises on my forehead to remind me that life can bring beauty in the most fragile moments. . . . Many people who are subject to seizures can have different perspectives on this condition: either their epilepsy is a burden or it is a bettering of their courage. I continue to uphold the latter of the choices."[4]

In March 2016, Gillian Mangan posted "An Elegy for Epilepsy" on her blog called *Gillian's Journey*, which in her words is "dedicated to my findings as a young adult overcoming this condition, and how the strength of others has reflected in my own strength." With her permission, her elegy follows:

Today, I was reminded by my body's limit to certain events. As I am only three months clear from my previous burst of seizures, I flutter around in my mind with wonderful possibilities of feeling included, of being welcomed with open arms to social soirees and smiling without a single worry. The explicit truth is that I *am* welcomed with opened arms. The scene that surrounds me is one of pure love and understanding, yet, there are moments where my body feels rather like a shell than a composition of wriggly fingers and toes. My mind can wander but, for now, my body cannot.

Epilepsy, I forgive you. You did not single me out in a room of young adults and say, "yes, that's the one that should have seven seizures in less than six weeks." Not your best idea, Epilepsy. However, I do not hold reality against you. Though I am restricted by your effect, I am not restricted by your presence in my spirit. I take into full account that you can hurt me and those whom I love the most, but I refuse to let you do so. My life will continue cautiously but excitingly, because you have opened doors for me. You have been a surprising conversation starter, a comfort to those who still stare at you with wide, terrified eyes. You bring me closer to *the* condition, not *my* condition. You have brought me closer to myself, to who I want to be.

The subject of one of my classes this week is narrowed around the demand of forgiveness. The scope is surrounded by forgiveness to not only those who have harmed us but also to those who we have harmed as well, specifying the concept of accepting ourselves in every unique form that we display. The unique forms are what we exude emotionally, our natural impulses in the exposed moments of life. Often, we are surprised by our uniqueness, taken aback by our own capabilities of honesty or gratitude.

Honestly, the reality of being restricted by my own body can be brutal at the split second of realization. Yet, the split second passes, the brutality is brushed over by forgiveness to the condition, and the entirety of the matter is minor in the dire circumstances. This is not a dire circumstance, nor will I let it be. Epilepsy, you make me want to save the dire circumstances. You are the point of reference to life's bigger matters, to cases that cannot be fathomed, written about, or spoken of. To those who live in fear of Epilepsy, find the silver lining. To live in fear of Epilepsy is to live in fear of yourself. Look at Epilepsy as a constant companion who reminds you that there is indeed glory in the small successes. Release the terror while you can and invest the emotion elsewhere, to a place that needs the attention more than a chronic diagnosis that can be dealt with. Find reason to empathize because of Epilepsy; we are all capable of moving beyond the standards of sympathy.[5]

## Who Can Drive and When

What teenager does *not* want to drive a car? Getting a driver's license is like a rite of passage, moving from one stage of life to another. Being able to drive provides a sense of freedom and independence. While teenagers whose seizures are controlled can drive safely and legally, the privilege of driving carries restrictions for some people who have epilepsy.

Nearly all states require individuals with epilepsy to be seizure-free for a certain time period before being allowed to drive. That time period can range from a few months to two years.

In Florida, for example, applicants and licensed drivers must be seizure-free for a period of two years before being approved for licensing. However, the law states that if an individual with epilepsy is under regular medical supervision, he or she may apply for a license at the end of a one-year seizure-free period. Illinois applicants with epilepsy will be granted a license if they submit a doctor's statement certifying that they can safely operate an automobile. There is no specific seizure-free period. New Yorkers with epilepsy must be seizure-free for one year before they can obtain a license and must submit a doctor's statement confirming this fact. The seizure-free period in Washington, DC, is one year. Californians with epilepsy must be seizure-free for three to six months before they can be issued a driver's license. Licensing laws can be found at each state's Department of Motor Vehicles.

In some cases, teenagers (and adults) continue to drive regardless of the risk of having seizures while on the road. Not surprisingly when seizures occur while driving, accidents happen, sometimes causing property damage and injuries to those with epilepsy as well as others. Drivers have to determine whether peoples' lives (including their own) are at risk if they ignore licensing laws.

## Seizure-Alert Dogs

Seizure-alert dogs—sometimes called support, assistant, or service dogs—have the ability to sense and alert a person with epilepsy that she or he is about to have a seizure. In recent years, news stories, magazine articles, YouTube videos, and Internet postings have described and occasionally shown what these dogs (and sometimes cats) do for their human friends.

The Epilepsy Foundation says seizure-alert dogs are like "an alarm system. They are helpers, protectors and service providers. So-called seizure response dogs can be all these things—and more." On its website, the foundation explains,

> A response dog might be trained to bark when a child has a seizure so that family members know what is happening. Or, a seizure dog may put its body in between the seizing individual and the floor to break the fall at the inception of a seizure. Some seizure dogs may even be trained to activate some kind of pre-programmed device such as a pedal that rings an alarm. . . . However, getting a dog with the special skill of recognizing seizures

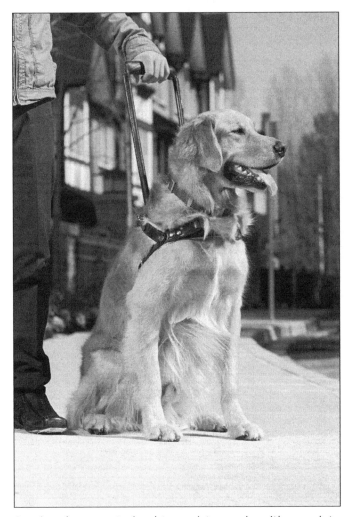

Service dogs are trained to assist people with a variety of ailments. Trained dogs can alert an epileptic individual up to an hour in advance of a seizure. ©iStock.com/XiXin Xing

in advance is another matter. Any claims by trainers that they can produce this type of behavior in a dog should be looked at very carefully, especially when the training is expensive. . . . More research is needed to better understand what dogs can and cannot do, whether there are differences between breeds, and how best to develop this unique skill.[6]

Several minutes before a seizure happens, a dog may bark, paw, or circle around its owner. A cat might howl or pace. A real-life video on YouTube shows a young woman with epilepsy and how her dog, Layla, recognizes that she is about to have a seizure. Layla alerts her by putting her head on the young woman's lap. Another video shows the woman having a seizure with Layla staying close by until her seizure is over.[7]

At times, when a person with an alert dog is in a public place, someone comes along and pets the dog, which creates a distraction. That situation happened to sixteen-year-old Hailey Ashmore in 2014. Her experience along with photographs are posted online. She was out and had her dog Flyyn, who was only seven months old, on a leash beside her. A "well-meaning" person came up to pet the dog, in spite of the large red patch with the word STOP on the dog's back. Because of the disruption, Flyyn did not sense that Hailey was about to have a seizure. Hailey fell and was injured. "I wish people could understand that's what the giant stop sign patch means," she says. "If somebody distracts him I can get seriously hurt. . . . If you see a service dog in public please educate your children, your friends, your family, anybody else that they are doing a really important job."[8]

Organizations such as Canine Partners for Life (CPL) train alert dogs, which takes at least two years. "Service dogs must be physically sound, temperamentally stable, happy working partners. Great care is taken to select only the most appropriate dogs for this level of work," CPL states on its website. The organization "uses primarily Labrador retrievers in its service dog program, but also utilizes golden retrievers, poodles, and labradoodles."[9]

Other experiences of people who have seizure-alert dogs appear in various media. The Texas *Lubbock Avalanche-Journal* published a story in 2014 titled "Dog Helps Teen Girl with Epilepsy Complete High School Education." The article explained that nineteen-year-old Jessica Hayes, with the help of her seizure-alert dog Shawnee, was able to attend Roosevelt High School classes for three years and get her diploma. Hayes, of Idalou, Texas, "started getting seizures when she was a freshman in high school, and before Shawnee, she was having two a week at times. Though not life-threatening, the seizures have caused a few black eyes and damage to Hayes's shoulders, resulting in 30 dislocations and four surgeries," the newspaper reported. Canine Partners for Life in Pennsylvania trained Shawnee and matched the dog with Hayes in 2011. "Shawnee can sense [Hayes's] seizures 10 to 15 minutes before they happen, and she sounds the alarm by jumping, glaring and disobeying commands. . . . This gives her time to call her parents and find a place to sit or lie down to prepare for what's coming." The alert dog and continued medication have helped Hayes achieve some independence and attend college (along with Shawnee).[10]

## Now You Know

- The Americans with Disabilities Act gives individuals with disabilities the right to have their service dogs with them in buildings, such as stores and courthouses, and in facilities like public bathrooms.

In 2016, *Fox 5 News* in Atlanta, Georgia, reported Rosalie Brown's story. Twenty-four-year-old Brown has epilepsy and unpredictable seizures. Some are so small that they are hardly noticeable, but they occur fifty to hundreds of times a day. Others are major and "violent." She told the news team that she has dislocated her shoulder many times during a seizure and has had to wear a sling for weeks. Until she got a seizure-alert dog in 2015, she could not go anywhere alone.

Brown had to wait four years for her furry helper, named Rolex. He came from Canine Assistants in Milton, Georgia, which trains dogs. Brown was asked to select one of two animals. But she did not make the decision. Rolex did. "He walked in, dragging his leash behind him. 'He kind of sniffed around,' Rosalie said. 'And then came directly up to me and picked up the end of his leash and handed it to me. And, he jumped in my lap and buried his head in my chest and would not move.'" They have been together ever since. "If Rosalie has a seizure, Rolex is trained to go alert the nearest person. He'll tug at their clothing, pulling them to Rosalie. He can also bring her the phone, or push a button that automatically dials 911," Beth Galvin of *Fox 5 News* reported.[11]

Another news story focused on Dezmond Hill of Albuquerque, New Mexico. Dezmond Hill was eighteen when Donna Olmsted of the *Albuquerque Journal* interviewed him in 2014. Hill "has multiple kinds of seizures . . . [but] has played sports, participated in Marine ROTC and worked hard academically." He has accomplished all of this with his alert dog Shadow at his side. "'It means a lot to have him. It means even if I'm alone, I'm still safe,'" Hill explain[ed] one day after basketball practice. 'He's my best friend. He's always there for me through thick and thin.'"[12]

"Dezmond Hill . . . created Paws for Epilepsy in September 2013 to help raise awareness and provide information and support for people with epilepsy and their families," Olmsted reported. "Through fundraising events he raises money to provide grants for families for service dogs and for equipment and devices that help keep people with epilepsy alive. Paws for Epilepsy is specifically raising money for grants for five New Mexico families for seizure response dogs and smart watches [wearable computing devices]."[13]

Seizure dogs are very expensive to train. An Ohio nonprofit agency called 4 Paws for Ability spends $22,000 to breed and train dogs and requests that each family raise $15,000 to cover expenses. Few people with epilepsy can afford to purchase them. But charitable organizations often raise funds for those who need these canine helpers.

# SCHOOL, WORK, AND DATING

*"My epilepsy hasn't really stopped me from doing things. I'm in 11th grade now at a public school. Most kids at my school don't even know I have epilepsy."*
—Kayla Brown on WebMD.com[1]

Along with changes in lifestyle and expectations, teenagers with epilepsy often must deal with uncertainty and anxiety about school and whether they will they be able to take part in most activities. A major concern is what others, especially friends and classmates, will think if they witness a seizure. They also wonder whether they will be accepted at social events and by coworkers if they have part-time or full-time jobs.

One teenager said that when her friends first learned about her epilepsy, they kept their distance for a while. When they got used to her seizures, they thought her behavior was rather amusing because once she got on top of her desk and began to act like she was swimming. She was teased about other seizure actions. She finally decided that some of her classmates were not true friends. Her real friends did not make fun of her and were supportive when she had seizures.

When people have mistaken ideas about epilepsy, their reactions to seizures can sometimes be cruel and demeaning. Some teenagers with epilepsy have reported instances of harassment, ridicule, and exclusion because they have had seizures in public. A mother in Florida said that when her son David was school-age, she had to defend him against neighborhood bullies who feared and harassed David and threatened the family.

Adults, too, have misconceptions about epilepsy. It is not unusual for school personnel to believe that a young person having a seizure is "faking it" or "acting crazy" in an attempt to gain attention. Numerous young people with epilepsy have been assigned to special education classes because teachers and other school personnel have wrongly concluded that epilepsy is akin to mental retardation.

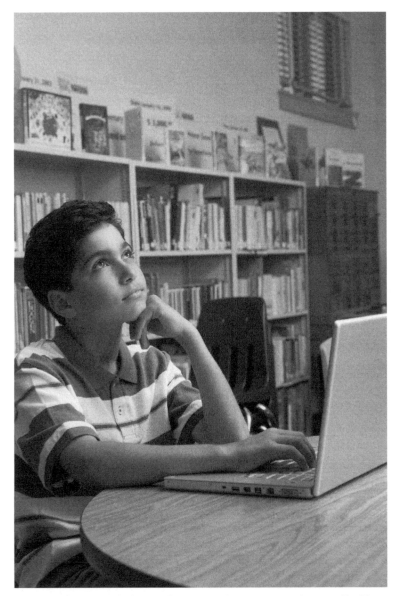

Some young people have absence seizures or staring spells. They stop what they are doing and stare vacantly for a few seconds, and then continue as if nothing happened.

Some people with mental retardation may have epilepsy, but epilepsy is not an intellectual problem. To repeat: Epilepsy is a brain disorder that causes seizures.

## Seizures in School

What happens when someone has a seizure in school? Those who have had that experience tell about it online and in news accounts. Sondra was thirteen years old when she reported, "I have the kind of epilepsy that makes me go rigid and then shake all over. The worst thing was having seizures at school and having to deal with everyone's reactions. I'm sure I looked totally weird. I was actually kind of relieved when I was told I had epilepsy because at least I knew what my problem was and could start taking medication for it."[2]

Consider Gemma. She had her first seizure when she was in a British middle school. She was interviewed when she was seventeen and described her experience on a video posted on the website HealthTalk.org.

> I had a pretty impressive [seizure] or faint off [at] the back of the Science stall. And we went to hospital then and . . . they didn't really know what was wrong, and basically said that I could go home. . . . And nothing really happened for another few years and then I started having blackouts. I'd faint. . . . I used to faint quite a lot. And at first we thought it was related to blood sugar. . . . And then we went to a different doctor who was a diabetes specialist and he said, "No that's wrong, it's nothing like that." And then he sent me to a neurologist by which time my seizures were getting a lot worse and I was having more major ones.[3]

Gemma had more seizures in school. She noted that one occurred in the common room where there were lockers.

> I had quite a major seizure . . . headfirst into the lockers, and I was totally out of it so I don't remember much of it. . . . At one point I thought I was going insane when I first sort of came around afterwards 'cos there was a vibrating by my head, which turned out to be my friend's phone 'cos I had also landed on her bag. But people were really supportive, there were people that sort of didn't know me that were . . . saying, "You okay?" . . . So it was really nice to know that even people that I don't necessarily know were being supportive.[4]

Gemma told HealthTalk.org that she planned to go to nursing school, and she would "not let epilepsy stand 'in her way to do anything she wants' and by taking a little more care, she can live her life as everyone else. . . . She doesn't think epilepsy has changed her sense of self because 'no medical condition defines who you are, it is just something you happen to have.'"[5]

A Rockford, Illinois, teen also had seizures while in school. Wesley Jones and his mother, Anita, decided he needed to change schools. Can a school make a difference in whether a student has seizures? Evidently, that is what happened. Jones told local *13 News* in 2016 that his seizures were "'probably just stress. The hallways were packed. Being around a lot of people set me off with a seizure,'" he explained.[6]

He transferred to LYDIA Urban Academy. "It's a non-traditional private school in downtown Rockford, where he's one of just 19 students," Kelsie Passolt of *13 News* reported. "Ever since he started going there, something remarkable has happened. 'He has not had one seizure in school since he's been here,' says LYDIA Urban Academy Director Chad Carty."[7] While at the academy, Wesley began a work-study program at the Epilepsy Foundation.

## Workplace Issues

It is common for teenagers with epilepsy to worry about getting a job and being able to keep working. They fear employers will not hire them or if on the job, they will have a seizure and be embarrassed, or worse, be fired.

The Americans with Disabilities Act (ADA; it was amended in 2008 and referred to as ADAA) prohibits discrimination against people with disabilities in employment, transportation, public accommodations, communications, and governmental activities. However, some people with epilepsy resent being classified as disabled. Nevertheless, the ADA protects against discrimination those who have seizures. The U.S. Equal Employment Opportunity Commission (EEOC) enforces the employment provisions of the ADA. It states that an employer may not ask a job applicant whether she or he has epilepsy, has seizures, uses prescription drugs, has filed for workers' compensation, or has been injured on the job. And applicants do not have to disclose that they have epilepsy.

There are instances when employers can ask about medical conditions. If, for example, they have a reasonable belief that employees may be unable to perform their jobs or may pose a direct threat to themselves or others. The employer may ask for medical information and obtain only the information needed to make an assessment of the employee's *present* ability to perform her or his job and to do so safely.

One example is cited by the EEOC: A newspaper reporter, who has been on leave for four months following experimental surgery for frequent seizures, notifies her employer that although she appears to be seizure-free, she will need to have follow-up appointments with her doctor for the next six months. Because the reporter's job frequently requires her to travel on short notice, the employer may ask her to provide a doctor's note indicating whether she can travel during the next six months and, if so, whether there are any limits on how long she can be away. (For a full explanation of the EEOC's enforcement of ADA for people with epilepsy, check the appendix.)

Employers also may ask employees about epilepsy when they have a reasonable belief that workers will be unable to safely perform the essential functions of their job because of epilepsy. In addition, an employer may ask an employee about

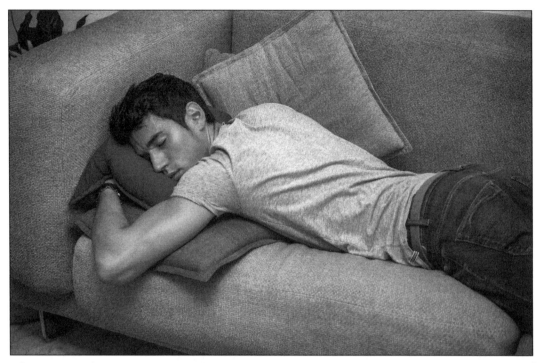

After a tonic clonic seizure (grand mal), a person may be very tired and confused. ©*iStock/ Art-Of-Photo*

epilepsy to support her or his request for a reasonable accommodation needed because of epilepsy; to verify the employee's use of sick leave related to epilepsy (for example, employees who have seizures sometimes sleep afterward for long periods); or to enable the worker to participate in a voluntary wellness program.

An employer may exclude an individual with epilepsy from a job for safety reasons when the individual poses a direct threat. A "direct threat" is a significant risk of substantial harm to the individual or others that cannot be eliminated or reduced through reasonable accommodation. This determination must be based on objective, factual evidence, including the best recent medical evidence and advances in the treatment of epilepsy. In making a direct threat assessment, the employer must evaluate the individual's present ability to safely perform the job

## Now You Know

● Studies show that workers with epilepsy and those without the disorder do not differ in accident and absenteeism rates and job performance. If there are safety concerns on the job, some simple accommodations may enable the person with epilepsy to perform the work effectively and safely.

by considering the duration of the risk; the nature and severity of the potential harm; the likelihood that the potential harm will occur; and the imminence of the potential harm.[8]

Samantha is one young adult who was removed from her job because of an epileptic seizure. According to Samantha, her employer's "excuse" was that she was at risk of harming herself should she have a seizure on her own. Samantha wrote, "I was forced to resign so they could fill my job. I remember crying to my boss, after 3 years of being a loyal employee I could not understand the lack of empathy that came from her, and to this day I still can't. I am very lucky to have gained a position with a unit that completely understands what I go through, empathizes with my situation, and provides anything they can to make it as easy as possible for me. For that, I cannot thank them enough."[9]

Another young adult with epilepsy faced difficulties when applying for a job, first with the U.S. Army (where he was turned down) and then as a state trooper. Using the name Strugglingtochasemydreams, he explained on Epilepsy.com in 2016 that he was eighteen years old with "controlled epilepsy and [had] been seizure free for a year by taking medication." He attended college for a year and achieved a 3.7 grade point average. Afterward, he wrote,

> [I] immediately sent an application in to the state troopers. I attended orientation, then passed my written exam with a 91. Then I took a physical test performing the 1.5 mile run in 10 minutes flat, 60 pushups in one minute, and 50 sit ups in one minute. Finally, I spent 3 days formatting all the official paperwork and documentation and in return I received an email about 3 weeks later saying that it was in my best interest not to pursue a career with the state troopers without them explaining why. However, I know why and it's because of my controlled epilepsy. All my attempts at finding a dream job whether it be with the army or the state troopers have been shot down.[10]

Still the young man did not give up. He became a volunteer fire fighter, hoping that would lead to a job with the police force.

## Dating

Worries about dating and dating issues are common among teenagers, whether or not they have epilepsy. But concerns intensify when there is the possibility of having a seizure in public or while on a date. One woman with epilepsy explained her experience to Peter Fox on Epilepsy.org.uk: "People were very quick to judge once they found out I have epilepsy. What many found even more strange was

## Epilepsy Bill of Rights

People living with epilepsy created a bill of rights for themselves and others who have seizures. "*The Bill of Rights for People Living with Epilepsy* is designed to inform people affected by epilepsy about issues related to healthcare, health insurance coverage, life at school and life in the workplace," according to Phylis Feiner Johnson on EpilepsyTalk.com. "People with epilepsy are encouraged to be their own advocates in managing their healthcare. However, any and all treatment decisions must be made together with their healthcare team." *The Bill of Rights for People Living with Epilepsy* is not a legal or medical document. It is a list of aspirations that the epilepsy community should try to achieve:

1. People with epilepsy have the right to be treated fairly and with respect.
2. People with epilepsy have the right to receive comprehensive, understandable information about epilepsy and its treatment.
3. People with epilepsy have the right and responsibility to be active members of their healthcare team.
4. People living with epilepsy have the right to know and understand all of the treatment options that are available to them.
5. Special populations of people with epilepsy (e.g., children, adolescents, women of child-bearing age, people with developmental disabilities, the elderly, etc.) have the right to ask about treatment and information appropriate to their specific needs.
6. People living with epilepsy have the right to understand all of the options and legal protections for accessing healthcare benefit coverage available to them.
7. People with epilepsy have the right to know that healthcare providers will hold personal and medical information confidential.
8. Children with epilepsy may have the right to receive special education and related services at school; parents have the right to advocate for such services.

9. People with epilepsy have the right to know that there are federal and state laws that may provide them with protections in the workplace.

10. People with epilepsy have the right to access help and support that will assist them in making informed decisions about living with epilepsy.[a]

that I couldn't drive. In the past couple of years, it has put men off dating me. I have been told I am 'different' or a 'liability.' I once didn't tell a young man I had epilepsy until the fourth date. He seemed very interested until I told him—then I never heard from him again. I was worried I would never find anyone who understands and isn't scared of epilepsy."[11]

Helen, who was age twenty-three when interviewed on HealthTalk.org about her dating experiences, noted,

I feel like I'd rather go out with someone that I know very well, or . . . at least know quite well because then the epilepsy for a start won't be more of a problem, they know more about me. I'd feel horrid about going out with someone, like on a first date, if I didn't know them very well. When

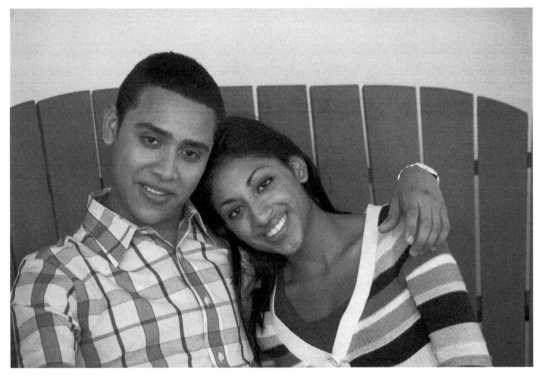

Many young people with epilepsy wonder when or if they should explain to a date that they have epilepsy.

do you bring it up? When do you tell them? What point do you tell someone that I have epilepsy? . . . And I think in that way it's . . . made me very afraid of getting involved in a relationship because you bring up a whole great heapful of things that you don't necessarily want to tell someone that you're not very involved with yet. . . .

I think it's changed the way that I think about relationships with people and I think the reason that I'd rather be friends with someone now before going out with them, is that I've kind of tested them, because you know at a certain point in my friendship with people it does come out. . . . So it has changed the way that I get involved in relationships a great deal and probably for the better. . . . You know it means that I'm a lot more picky. But it is good.[12]

Twenty-one-year-old Finlay was also interviewed for HealthTalk.org. He said, "Most of the girls I've been out with have been okay" with his epilepsy. "I'd rather be friends with someone now before going out with them . . . you know at

## What Young Women with Epilepsy Say

On the website GirlswithNerve.com, young women tell what they encounter when they inform people that they have epilepsy. Stephanie said, "I've had people walk away when I said I have epilepsy. Even when I try to explain that I'm still a normal functioning person. When that happens, at first I feel kind of hurt. But then I come to realize that if a person is going to judge someone based on a condition that they didn't choose to have, then they aren't good enough for me."

Another young woman, Alexandra, said, "I don't believe in sugarcoating anything. If someone wants to be an important part of my life, they can't be wary of me because of my epilepsy. When I tell people about my epilepsy, I just straight up tell them, 'Hey I do have epilepsy, here's what to do if I have a seizure.'"

Ashley said, "I have made an informational video about epilepsy that I put on Facebook. I get all my friends to watch it. It helped all my friends because I think people should know right away what you have. It's being caught by surprise that seems to make people scared."[b]

a certain point in my friendship with people it does come out. It just comes out, why don't I drive? Why don't I drink? I tell them and if I've known for a while then they have kind of passed the test . . . then I don't mind going out with them. I've got much less to lose. . . . I don't like to go out with people who would be awkward talking about [epilepsy], because I'm not awkward talking about it."[13]

# SPORTS AND RECREATION

..................................................................................................

*"It's probably for my best health not to play football anymore."*
—*lineman Boo Simon, who was recruited for the University of South Florida football team,*
*but declined to play due to his epileptic seizures*[1]

Most people with controlled seizures can take part in a variety of sports, recreational activities, and physical training. Team and individual sports play an important role in the lives of many young people with epilepsy. Even a person who has seizures once a week may take part in sports and recreation. After all, there are still many days when that person is seizure-free.

Certainly some risks also have to be avoided. People with epilepsy are advised not to take part in such sports as motor racing, skydiving, hang gliding, scuba diving, recreational flying, and other activities that require concentration at all times. Mountain climbing can pose hazards as well. Reduced oxygen and atmospheric changes at some elevations may increase the risks of seizures.

Recreational activities such as bicycling, swimming, boating, and horseback riding are relatively safe for a person who has seizures, but precautions should be taken, such as wearing a helmet while bicycling or horseback riding, alerting a lifeguard before swimming, and boating only with another person along.

Whether taking part in individual or team sports or recreational activities, athletes with epilepsy are at risk of seizures if they refuse or forget to take their antiepileptic drugs. That is exactly what happened to a teenager treated by Elaine Wyllie, MD. In an article for *U.S. News and World Report*, Dr. Wyllie wrote in 2015 that her patient, a fifteen-year-old boy, who had epilepsy, was "an outstanding" athlete and "loved to play football. . . . But suddenly, in late middle school, his seizures increased. He was experiencing grand mal, or generalized tonic-clonic, seizures with whole-body jerky movements and unawareness for two to three minutes followed by a recovery period, with sleepiness and confusion for up to 30 minutes. His parents and coaches became concerned, and reluctantly they

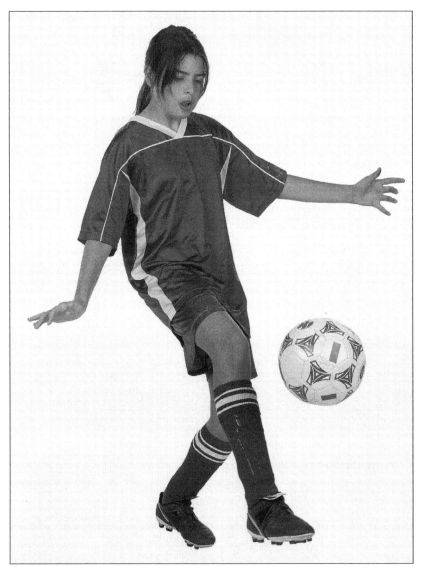

Young people with epilepsy can safely take part in some team sports.

delivered the news that for his own safety, he should stop playing."[2] However, doctors at Cleveland (Ohio) Clinic's Epilepsy Center learned that the teenager had stopped taking his medication because it was making him nauseated. Dr. Wyllie prescribed a different medication with a promise from the young athlete that he would follow directions.

"Research shows that up to half of patients with epilepsy may not take their medications as directed," Wyllie noted, "and this is especially true for teenagers. The medical term for this is non-adherence, and among people who present to emergency rooms because of increased seizures, it is the cause of the increase in over 50 percent of cases."[3]

Boo Simon is one person with epilepsy who took his medications and as a teenager had a promising career in football. When he was senior at Alabama's Baldwin County High, the six-foot-four, 280-pound offensive lineman signed with the University of South Florida. But before the 2012 college season began, he had seizures during practice and drills. Some of them were minor but others were violent. Simon decided to drop out after learning he had epilepsy. "I don't have the scary epilepsy. . . . I can tell when it's coming. I can feel it coming probably an hour before it happens." Nevertheless, he decided he "had to walk away from the game. I know some players have been able to play with [epilepsy]. But, I think my life, my brain is more important down the road than football," he told Josh Bean of the Alabama Media Group.[4]

## It Happened to Jessica

In the May 2011 issue of *American Cheerleader*, Jessica Waters of Beavercreek, Ohio, was the focus of a cover story about her life with epilepsy. The article is titled "I Have Epilepsy; It Doesn't Have Me." When she was in elementary school, Jessica's teachers had reported that Jessica was daydreaming a lot. But Jessica was having multiple seizures a day and could not remember what happened at school.

The article describes how Jessica, at age eleven, struggled with anger and depression after neurologists at Dayton Children's Hospital diagnosed her epilepsy. Her parents Scott Register and Chastity Irwin credit a nurse in the neurology department at the hospital for helping their daughter turn her life around.

As a teenager, Jessica became a cheerleader for Beavercreek City Schools, a member of the varsity dance team, and a volunteer at an epilepsy camp for children. Jessica also was named Junior Teen America 2012. She is the founder of the nonprofit Cupcakes for Camp, whose "mission is to educate the public about epilepsy . . . and to send kids to camp so they can enjoy being a kid. Lastly to encourage teens to volunteer and to make volunteering 5 hours required for graduation."

Jessica has this advice for teenagers: "If you know someone with epilepsy, listen and be their friend. And to all the kids with epilepsy, we will beat this together or at least help each other through the hard days. You have epilepsy, but it doesn't or won't ever have you."[a]

# Famous Athletes with Epilepsy

Athletes who have epilepsy and have become famous in team and individual sports are often an inspiration to young and aspiring players who are prone to seizures. Famous athletes inspire by what they have accomplished in sports. Here are some selected examples:

Pittsburgh Steelers right guard Alan Faneca started having seizures when he was fifteen years old. Nevertheless, he continued to play football in high school, college, and finally with the Steelers; he played his final game at the end of the 2010 season. Faneca's daughter also has epilepsy, and since his retirement, Faneca has helped educate the public about epilepsy.

Jason Snelling is another former football player who was diagnosed with epilepsy. He was twenty years old at the time, and became involved with the Epilepsy Foundation while in college. A defensive back for the Atlanta Falcons for seven years, Snelling retired in 2014. He often speaks out and encourages young athletes at various epilepsy-awareness events.

Davis Tarwater is an American swimmer and Olympic gold medalist. He was diagnosed with epilepsy as a young child growing up in Knoxville, Tennessee. He began to compete in swimming at age seven. During his teenage years, he set three state swimming records and led his high school to the state title. He was named High School Swimmer of the Year in 2002.

Olympic silver medalist Marion Clignet is a French American athlete with many titles for international and national cycling races. She was diagnosed with epilepsy in 1986 at the age of twenty-two. Because of her seizures she could not drive, so bicycling was her means of transportation. That led to her interest in competitive cycling and ultimately her awards.

Mike Simmel, known as "Mighty Mike," was a member of the famous Harlem Wizards basketball team from 2001 to 2014. The Wizards entertain by using a variety of basketball tricks and comedy. Simmel began having atonic seizures as a youngster. During his teen years and as an adult, he has had petit mal and tonic-clonic seizures, but has been able to control them and serve as a national spokesman for epilepsy.

Ice hockey athlete Chanda Gunn was a goalie for the 2006 U.S. Olympic team. She was diagnosed with epilepsy at the age of nine. As an adult she not only enjoys ice hockey as a sport, but also is an activist for epilepsy awareness programs.

David "Dai" Greene is a British hurdler who has epilepsy. He was taking medications to control his seizures, and while in college was out with his friends on a Friday night. "'I was a typical college student—it was all about drinking, playing sport and having fun,'" he told the *Daily Mail*, a U.K. newspaper. "The last thing I remember, I was with my mates in the pub. And then my mum was picking me up and putting me to bed. I'd had a [seizure]. I was unconscious and convulsing, although I didn't know it at the time. I know what a convulsion looks like because my brother has epilepsy, too, and it isn't very nice to watch."[5] After more seizures, Greene eventually changed his lifestyle, stopped drinking, ate healthy food, and got more sleep. He went on to win the 400 meter hurdles at the European Championships in Barcelona in 2010 and the World Championship gold in the 400 meter hurdles in 2011.

## Summer Camps

During the summer, camps offering a variety of recreational and sports activities for young people with epilepsy are conducted in various parts of the United States. While some of the camps are geared toward preteens, others are for teenagers and young adults. For example, in Colorado, the Jason Fleishman Summer Camp is located in Estes Park. "It is a five-day overnight camp for teens living with epilepsy. The camp provides an opportunity for young people with epilepsy to participate in fun and exciting activities like rock climbing, zip line, horseback riding, arts and crafts and more," the Epilepsy Foundation reports. It is "a safe, medically monitored setting."[6]

Other Epilepsy Foundation–sponsored camps include Channel 3 Kids Camp for ages eight to twenty-one "by the shores of the Skungamaug River, in Andover and Coventry, CT. There are more than 25 buildings that include sleeping cabins, an open air pavilion, dining hall, recreation hall, arts & crafts cabin . . . swimming pool and more." The cost was $295 in 2016.

In Illinois, Camp Blackhawk is a week-long retreat for young people ages six to seventeen who have epilepsy. "There is NO cost to attend camp, however, donations are accepted and welcomed. . . . Space is limited and campers are accepted on a first-come, first-serve basis." The Greater Chicago area affiliate gives priority to people within their service area.

Camp Oz in Minnesota offers "a weeklong overnight camp for youth and teens [ages nine to seventeen] whose primary condition is epilepsy. It's a great opportunity for youth to experience a safe yet fun camping experience that includes swimming, horseback riding, campfires, games, sports, nature and meeting new friends." Campers paid $300 to attend in 2016.

In Pennsylvania, "Camp Achieve is a week-long overnight camp for children and teens with epilepsy/seizure disorder." Organized and operated by the Eastern Pennsylvania affiliate of the Epilepsy Foundation, the camp serves young people ages eight to seventeen. "The week is a time for building independence, making friends and learning how to manage a life with seizures and just having fun!" In 2016, the cost for the camp was $350 and scholarships were available.

## Mighty Mike

Basketball great Mike Simmel's middle-grade book *Mighty Mike Bounces Back* (Magination Press, 2011) is actually based on Simmel's experiences with epilepsy. In a section of the book titled "A Note from Mighty Mike," he writes:

> Like the Mighty Mike in the story, I once had major epileptic seizures in a basketball camp. I was 16, and my family and I refused to let the camp send me home. Obstacles like that one made me stronger. As a teenager my seizures came back and continued right through my adult years. Currently, I continue to take medication for my epilepsy and follow a physician's care. . . . I continued to work hard to develop my basketball skills, and I kept thinking positively. . . . I also got creative and developed more and more tricks that I could do with a basketball.[b]

The Coelho Epilepsy Youth Summer Camp in Occidental, California, enrolls youth ages six to seventeen. The camp provides young people ages nine to seventeen a variety of activities, including swimming, canoeing, archery, arts and crafts, gaga ball, going to the beach, hiking, sports, a talent show, tie-dye, and campfires. Medical professionals specializing in epilepsy care provide around the clock support. In 2016, the cost to attend the one-week camp was $625.

## Safe Recreation and Exercise

People with epilepsy can safely engage in most sports, even if they have occasional seizures. But if a person has severe seizures, he or she needs to limit or modify athletic activities, experts advise. Robert S. Fisher, MD, a professor of neurology at Stanford University, explains,

> All too often, families or medical advisors of people with epilepsy place a heavy blanket of restrictions over all activities that may even remotely lead to an injury. While reasonable precautions, like not allowing someone with uncontrolled seizures to fly a plane, are sensible . . . excessive restrictions

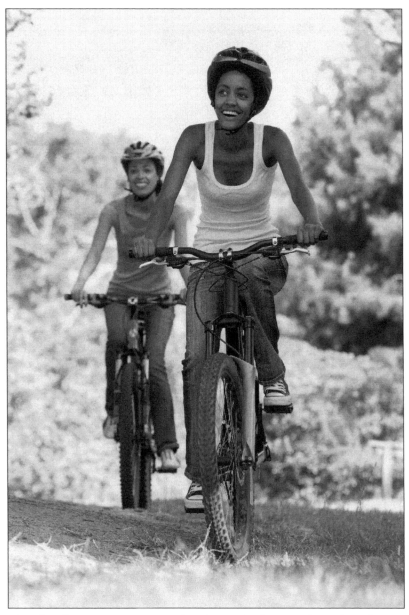

Bicycling is a common recreational activity for people with epilepsy.

can take the fun out of life and further stigmatize a person with epilepsy. . . . Some popular low risk activities are: running, bowling, golf, baseball, basketball, soccer, and volleyball. Medium risk activities, meanwhile, may be engaged in if seizures are mild or infrequent. . . . Some medium risk activities include football, hockey and ice skating, bike racing, gymnastics, horseback riding, swimming in shallow water with a buddy, and boating. . . . High-risk recreational activities include: hang gliding, motor sports. . . . At the very least, a patient should not participate in high risk recreation unless he or she has been seizure-free for years.[7]

## Read This!

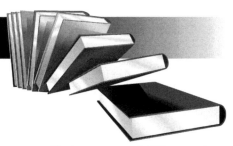

*The Islands at the End of the World* by Austin Aslan (Wendy Lamb Books/Random House, 2014) is set in Hawai'i, and in the opening pages the narrator, Leilani, is surfing the big waves off the coast of Hilo on the Big Island where she lives. She is "surfing to forget the EKGs and MRIs and OMGs" that she will be facing.[c] This is a hint that Leilani has epilepsy, which is confirmed a short time later. But the book is not just about Leilani's epilepsy. It is also about Leilani being a hapa, part native Hawaiian—her mother and grandparents are "pure Hawaiian," while her father is haole (white), a biology professor and avid conservationist. The family has moved to Hawai'i from California, and Leilani finds out what it is like to be bullied by high school classmates who have contempt for anyone not of Hawaiian heritage.

Leilani's heritage and her love for surfing and rock climbing are part of the background of the story. So is her epilepsy. In the early part of the story, Leilani and her father fly to the island of O'ahu, about forty minutes away, where she will take part in a clinical trial to determine the efficacy of antiseizure medications.

While in O'ahu Leilani has a seizure at the clinic and many tonic-clonic episodes afterward as she and her dad experience what appears to be a global nuclear fallout or some weird atmospheric happening that no one can understand. Electricity fails and all electronics shut down. The two are in for a wild adventure trying to get back to Hilo. One catastrophe after another—lack of transportation, food shortages, military oppression, riots, murders—prevents them from leaving O'ahu. Stress and angst cause Leilani to have numerous seizures, which she calls "fits" (an outdated term).

Leilani's father is by her side when she has seizures and, in the story, uses a "bite stick, a wooden tongue depressor that keeps the airways clear,"[d] which in the real world is considered dangerous and should never be used, according to epilepsy experts. As the story progresses, Leilani's epilepsy holds a clue to the disaster, and during her seizures she appears to be part of the Hawaiian mythology, native language, and culture.

Exercising is an important activity for almost everyone. But the Epilepsy Foundation has posted guidance for those who experience seizures. The Foundation's advice follows:

Most individuals with epilepsy can safely exercise in a gym, use exercise equipment, and do other types of exercise. A few thoughts:

For those who have uncontrolled seizures, use a buddy system. Especially when using equipment such as treadmills, weights, or even bike riding.

When riding a bike, avoid busy streets. Try bike paths or quiet residential streets instead. Don't forget the helmet!

Walking is even easier and doesn't cost anything. Use the same ideas— avoid busy streets and walk with a buddy.

Start small and don't tackle long periods of exercise right away!

Take frequent breaks and drink plenty of fluids.

If you tire easily, exercise in small amounts. Even 15 to 20 minutes at a time helps!

Always wear a medic alert bracelet or necklace and carry a medic alert card!

Look at seizure alert systems that are being developed. Using one with a GPS locator is a great idea in case you have a seizure and need help.

A cell phone with GPS locator can help people find you too! Program emergency numbers and key family members or contacts into your phone![8]

# FEMALE ISSUES

*"It's August, 2015 and I have been seizure free for two years! I am very interested in helping get the word out about epilepsy and I would like to help raise awareness."*
—Dani, communications adviser for GirlswithNerve[1]

More than one million U.S. women of child-bearing age have a seizure disorder. Females seem to cope with epilepsy differently than males, numerous experts say. Teen girls, for example, sometimes feel guilty about their disorder but may try to get help from parents or guardians. Boys, on the other hand, may try to be "macho" and attempt to hide any appearance of a disorder. Even if both genders deal with epilepsy in similar ways, there is no doubt that certain epilepsy issues are germane to females.

Females with epilepsy face more complex health care issues than do males with seizure disorders. Studies have shown that women may experience more frequent seizures around the time of their menstrual periods. Antiseizure medications, or antiepileptic drugs (AEDs) as they are often called, may also interfere with hormone regulation and can reduce the effectiveness of birth control pills. Seizures can harm not only a pregnant woman, but also her fetus. Seizures that cause a loss of consciousness and violent, jerking movements, are especially hazardous during pregnancy.

"Not only do they [women] have to cope with seizures, they must also deal with the impact the disorder can have on their reproductive health," states WebMD.com. "Epilepsy and seizure medications may affect contraception, pregnancy, and hormone levels, and the female reproductive cycle. . . . Many seizure drugs can prevent birth control pills from working effectively, which can lead to an unplanned pregnancy. . . . Women who are taking seizure medications should be especially careful about taking a multivitamin and extra folic acid." They are advised to check with their doctor about dosage "because some epilepsy medications deplete the body of important vitamins, particularly folic acid."[2]

## Birth Control

In some cases birth control for young women with epilepsy can be a complex matter. Amanda, a twenty-year-old attending New Jersey City University, wrote on August 29, 2015,

> On top of managing my medical needs with my epilepsy, I also had a difficult time trying to figure out my birth control. In 2014, I discovered I was getting severe pains on both my right and left ovaries, and I found out from my gynecologist that I had multiple cysts on both of my ovaries. I tried many different types of birth control, but I had issues with my menstrual cycle, insurance, and other things. A year later, 2015, I decided to stop using hormonal birth control, which was the best option for me. My advice for girls getting frustrated with not being able to find the right kind of birth control is to be patient even when times get tough.[3]

Amanda suggested linking to http://girlswithnerve.com/birth-control/, which discusses concerns such as birth control options, how birth control affects AEDs, hormonal birth control like the pill, and intrauterine devices.

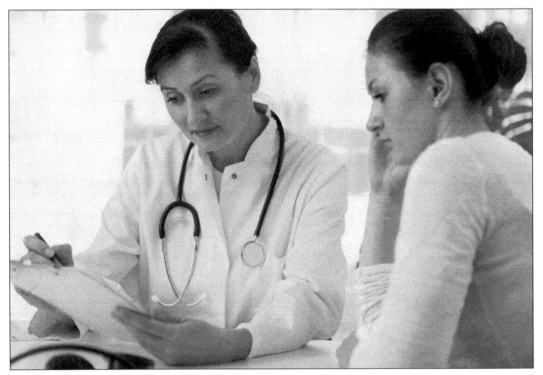

Young women with epilepsy who are pondering birth control options should consult a doctor. ©iStock.com/AlexRaths

Kristy explained on HealthTalk.org, "I'm not allowed to have any contraception, apart from condoms" because her seizures were not yet controlled. She explained, "My epilepsy is quite bad at the moment and [doctors] are waiting until it's controlled because the contraceptive pill will interfere with my lamotrigine [her AED] so I have to wait."[4]

## Sex and Pregnancy Concerns

It is not unusual for young women with epilepsy to worry about pregnancy or even whether to have intercourse. What if she has a seizure during sex? Doctors say there is no more likelihood that a seizure will occur during sex than at any other time. Rather, it is worry and stress that might trigger a seizure.

Women also wonder if they should ever have children. Even if they don't have epilepsy, maybe a partner does. Would that mean that their child might inherit a seizure disorder? Or women might be concerned that if they become parents, they will have seizures and endanger their children while caring for them.

Some young women with epilepsy believe they will never be able to have children, or they have been advised by relatives, friends, or even their doctors not to get pregnant because their children may suffer birth defects, such as autism. They may be alarmed by reports from women who say they would like to have a child one day but they worry about the side effects their antiseizure medication could have on a child. Yet, most women who have epilepsy give birth to healthy babies.

When twenty-year-old Carole was interviewed for HealthTalk.org, she said, "I've always known that I wanted children." But she added, "I did get told that . . . being epileptic I was at higher risk of having an autistic child, but I think it was only slightly, but that still brought concern to me."[5]

Canadian Heather Yade Girardin was worried about epilepsy for most of her life. Her mother had the disorder and died when Heather was only eight years old. She wrote on a Canadian website, EpilepsyStories.com, "I had been suffering my seizures on a regular basis for almost 2 years." After ruling out heart disease and other health problems, she and her boyfriend, now her husband, consulted a neurologist who diagnosed Heather's epilepsy.

Heather was sixteen when she got pregnant. After her child was born, Heather completed high school and cared for her daughter, even though her "seizures were a regular occurrence at the time varying in severity." Her son was born in 2009, and at that point, Heather "started on a low dose of medication. It helped reduce my number of seizures. A year later I went to college and graduated as a personal support worker." She has had seizures at work, but she wrote in 2015 that she was "returning to school for nursing" and planned to "continue working part time and raise [her] kids." Even though "fear and daunting" are always there, she declared, "With the support from family and friends I don't stop myself from having a full plate in life."[6]

Elana Gartner expressed her fears about becoming a mom in a post on Kvellar.com. Gartner explained that because she had epilepsy, she planned to adopt. "This was compounded by the fact that I was on a medication that was high-risk to take while pregnant." She decided that under the care of her doctor she would adjust her medications during a transition period before she and her husband would attempt to get pregnant. (It is important to get the balance of antiepileptic medication before pregnancy, which usually means reducing antiseizure drugs and allowing time for the body to adjust to the new levels.) Gartner wrote,

> My greatest fear in life, until that point, was that I would have a seizure. The medicine transition was like walking through fire; I was petrified. I had been seizure-free for five years. . . . The five-week transition went smoothly and, eight months later, we were allowed to start trying. . . . When we got pregnant, we worked with a high-risk OBGYN [obstetrician-gynecologist] at the same hospital as my neurologist.[7]

When the Gartners' son was born, Elana felt she had conquered her fears. But not long afterward she had a seizure. As she explained, "I had re-started my birth control several weeks earlier; it had crossed with the new medication and I was sleep-deprived from an emergency room visit the night before with my son."[8]

The Gartners had another child, a daughter, but Elana had not discussed her epilepsy with her children. "While writing this article, I finally found my courage and explained my epilepsy to my 4-year-old in age-appropriate terms," she reported. "I was stunned by how easily he took the news, the questions he asked (if during a seizure my brain didn't work a little, did that mean I was dead?) and how safe I suddenly felt, having told him."[9]

## Proper Medical Care

All women who become pregnant should get proper medical care early in their pregnancies. And any female of childbearing age with epilepsy should consult her obstetrician or family physician as soon as possible if she is pregnant, experts say. An important factor in childbearing is not the epilepsy itself, but the medication taken to control seizures.

Antiseizure medication should be taken during pregnancy, but some drugs can increase the risk of birth defects. A doctor can change antiseizure medications if necessary. In addition, vitamin supplements, particularly folic acid, can

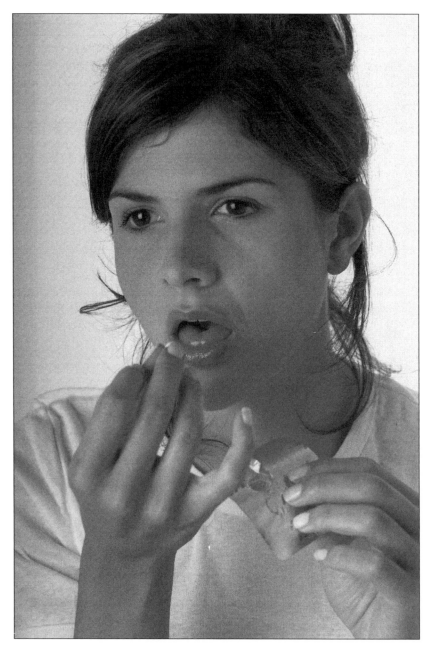

It is important that pregnant females with epilepsy take their pre-scribed antiseizure medication.

be started, reducing risks of birth defects. With prenatal counseling, a doctor can explain other health risks, such as the possibility of a premature birth, miscarriage, injury to a fetus during a seizure, or even stillbirth.

In addition, medical personnel often advise new moms with epilepsy to get help at home with a first baby. Stress, lack of sleep while caring for a newborn, and anxiety about child care could trigger seizures. Helpers can monitor and help protect new moms and their babies.

## Hormonal Changes

Hormonal changes, particularly during the teenage years, can have a direct effect on someone with epilepsy. Hormones are chemical substances in the body secreted from endocrine glands. They control or influence such processes as muscle growth, heart rate, behavior, the reproductive system, and the menstrual cycle. During puberty, hormones stimulate body changes that may have an effect on certain types of seizures. Some seizures that begin in childhood may disappear at puberty, while other types may begin at this time of hormonal changes.

The connection between seizures and hormones is not yet well understood. But according to WebMD.com, "Women with epilepsy face different issues than men with epilepsy. For some women, the pattern of epileptic seizures is directly affected by the normal hormonal cycles they experience throughout their lives. Two primary sex hormones flow through women's bodies. One is estrogen and the other is progesterone." Usually the female body has equal amounts of each hormone. But "both of these hormones interact with brain cells. Estrogen is an 'excitatory' hormone, which means that it makes brain cells give off more of an electrical discharge. Progesterone, on the other hand, is an 'inhibitory' hormone, which means that it calms those cells down. When the body is making more estrogen than progesterone, it can make the nervous system 'excitable.' In other words, [there is] a greater risk for seizures. The hormones aren't actually *causing* the seizures, but they can influence when they happen."[10]

Some females with epilepsy have seizures that are exacerbated by their menstrual cycle. It is a condition called catamenial epilepsy in which seizure frequency and severity are related to the level of certain reproductive hormones in the blood. "The exact cause of these seizures is unknown. However, some women have most of their seizures when there is a lot of estrogen in their body, such as during ovulation. Other women have seizures when progesterone levels tend to drop, such as right before or during their period," according to WebMD.com.[11]

## Birth Rates

Some reported studies contend that women with epilepsy have lower birth rates than those in the general population. Doctors at Medscape.com wrote that "lower birth rates in women with epilepsy may be due to social inhibitions. There may be fear of rejection due to seizures during social occasions, development of relationships, or intercourse. Fear of effects of epilepsy or its treatments on a pregnancy may cause women with epilepsy to seek contraception, abortions, and even sterilization." However, the Medscape doctors also noted that other research suggests

# Read This!

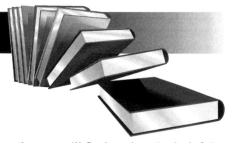

*The Sacred Disease: My Life with Epilepsy* by Kristin Seaborg, MD (Booktrope, 2015; Amazon Publishing, 2016), is a paperback and e-book that most females—teens, young adults, mothers—will find authentic, helpful, and inspirational. Others should read it too, primarily because so few nonepileptic individuals understand epilepsy. As Dr. Seaborg noted on a blog she started to raise awareness of epilepsy, "Although epilepsy is astoundingly common and strikingly prevalent, I am surprised every day about how *uncommon* it is for people to talk about epilepsy and how much stigma is still associated with this disease."[a]

Dr. Seaborg is a practicing pediatrician in Madison, Wisconsin, where she lives with her husband, Andrew, and their three children. Her book is a memoir and records her experiences with epilepsy, which was not diagnosed until she was eighteen years old, but began with her first seizure as a toddler. She noted in a 2012 post on her blog *One in Twenty-Six,*

> My first seizure, which lasted over 30 minutes, left a scar deep in my brain that served as a starting point for my future seizures. The complex partial seizures, or seizures that only involve part of my brain, that I have had since adolescence frequently sneak up and dance around the edges of my consciousness, stealing slivers of my alertness just enough to leave me tired and spent after 15–30 seconds of involuntary swallowing and clenching of my left hand. And although the partial seizures are subtle enough that only those closest to me would know something was amiss, they leave me feeling as if I have been battered, bruised, and in a fog for the rest of the day. I have learned to hide my symptoms as much as possible. In a world where there are still many misconceptions about seizures and Epilepsy, I find others squirming uncomfortably when I confess that I continue to have uncontrolled seizures. I notice colleagues changing the subject quickly when I mention Epilepsy. Anytime I feel the characteristic aura of a looming seizure, I search for a safe place to sit and hide in case the simple seizure generalizes into something more.[b]

Seaborg's book is in three parts: "The Student," "The Patient," and "The Mother"—all of her roles as someone with epilepsy. She describes her plans to become a physician and her fears that her seizures would prevent her from practicing medicine. In 2003, she had surgery to remove the area of her brain that had been damaged during infancy, but her seizures returned five months later. In one excerpt from her book, Seaborg describes a seizure that happened just before she was due to deliver her second child and she went outdoors for a walk:

> I walked and listened to the familiar music of the leaves and the trees when an aura swiftly materialized. *I told you so*, Epilepsy seemed to taunt through the pulsing heat and confusion, *you can't deny that I am a part of you.*
>
> I saw Andrew at the other end of the driveway and walked to him slowly through the developing seizure. Later, Andrew told me that I walked to him with a blank stare and stood quietly before I abruptly became rigid. My unconscious body slumped into his arms and he carefully lowered me to the ground just as the jarring muscle contractions of the seizure began.
>
> Andrew dragged my pregnant, convulsing body into the safety of our garage with effort. He placed my bobbing head on a pillow of recycled newspapers before he ran into the house to call 9-1-1.[c]

Happily, the Seaborgs' healthy eight-pound, four-ounce son, William, was born the next day. There is much, much more about the doctor's life and her uplifting messages on her blog and in her book. As an advocate for an epilepsy cure, all the royalties from Seaborg's book are donated to CURE (Citizens United for Research in Epilepsy).

---

that there is little difference in birth rates of women with seizure disorders and those who do not have epilepsy.[12]

Conclusions of a yearlong study titled "Women with Epilepsy: Pregnancy Outcomes and Deliveries" were published in *Clinical Neurology News* in April 2016. Participants in the study were "89 women with epilepsy and 109 healthy [women] who were seeking to become pregnant and had stopped using contraception within 6 months of enrollment or were about to stop using it." The study found that "live births occurred in 82% of pregnancies of women with epilepsy

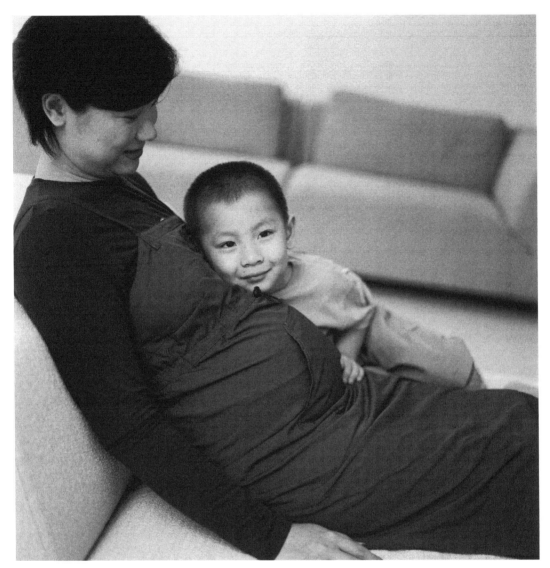

It is not unusual for pregnant women who have seizures to worry about whether they will be able to care for their children. But they often manage quite well.

and 80% of controls, while miscarriages occurred in 13% and 20%, respectively. Both of those rates are very similar to the general population."[13]

In a reaction to the study, Dr. Katherine Noe, an epilepsy specialist at the Mayo Clinic in Scottsdale, Arizona, praised the "first solid evidence" that the ability of women with epilepsy "to achieve pregnancy was no different than what was reported by a control population without epilepsy."[14]

# IMPACTS OF EPILEPSY ON FAMILIES

····································································································

*"You know, people with epilepsy may not say anything because they're afraid of how others will treat them. You can help change things by talking about it."*
—*Actress Hayden Panettiere on TalkaboutIt.com*[1]

When a family member has a seizure and gets a diagnosis of epilepsy, parents, siblings, and others often experience dread, frustration, and confusion. They also feel helpless. Parents who witness their child's seizure for the first time say the experience can be extremely frightening and shocking.

One thirteen-year-old girl had her first seizure followed by four others within a short time, and her mother said she had never been as frightened as she was on that day. She thought her child might die, but as the seizures subsided, she realized that she had to get medical help for her daughter.

Actor and film producer Harrison Ford, whose daughter has epilepsy, noted on TalkaboutIt.org, "There is a history of epilepsy in my family. I am really aware of what a devastating affliction it can be. It not only affects the person who suffers from epilepsy but it affects their entire family. It's really important to talk about it and find out about it. There's real important cutting edge research going on in the area and I'm very hopeful that someday very soon we'll find a cure for this really devastating affliction."[2]

## Frightening Impacts

J. R. McGarrahan, a retired army officer, described his reaction when his teenage son Sean had his first seizure one morning while both were reading the Sunday newspaper:

I heard a loud vocal sound, not a yell or shout, just an indistinct cry like a very noisy yawn coming from across the room. I looked over and saw Sean in a rigid position in the midst of a convulsion across the chair. He was shaking though not violently, and he did not seem to be aware of what he was doing. Soon he was lying on the floor, now moving around slightly erratically and gasping for air. As I first went over to him and talked to him, he really did not seem to be aware of me. I continued trying to talk with him, and soon he began to respond, but as if only half awake. That is, he seemed to know I was talking to him but really could not make sense of the words.

Meanwhile, his mother had come into the room and I asked her to call 911 for an ambulance. The five or fewer minutes of this experience seemed like hours on one hand yet like just seconds—all at the same time. My military experience kept my thoughts riveted on trying to "do something," even though I did not know exactly what. My heart, though, was saying "What is happening to my son?!" I had never seen someone experience a seizure before, so a sense of great concern jumped in quickly on top of being mystified.

Fortunately, fear of him dying from this episode came and went quickly as he regained fuller awareness of where he was and began breathing more normally. So fear, then mystery, then concern, then questions, then different concerns all swirled around in me as we waited.[3]

On HealthTalk.org, a woman in her twenties described her family's reaction to her seizures:

I think I've affected everyone. When I was in hospital everyone was really stressed out. . . . They were like they gave up. My sister, she couldn't eat, she couldn't sleep and the whole family was under stress. And my husband he was really stressed out, and my older son who was six and a half. . . . He was like crying all the time. And my younger one he was really attached to me before, but now he's more attached to my sister because she's been looking after him for over a year now. So he's more attached to her and my mother now.[4]

On the same website, one man with epilepsy explained his family's reactions. He said, "My grandparents, my grandmother particularly was really distraught, sobbing. . . . And basically my parents were supportive but, they kept . . . the lid on things. Yeah . . . there was a degree of shame. . . . I think they meant well and they were very supportive to me. But they didn't want to go round saying 'Excuse

## Photosensitivity

Photosensitive epilepsy is a condition in which moving or flickering lights can trigger a seizure. In today's world, these flickering lights may come from such sources as computer monitors, video games, television, strobe lights, fluorescent tubes, and even sunlight reflecting on water. Less than 5 percent of people with epilepsy today are photosensitive, and the frequency of flashing light that may provoke a seizure varies from person to person. Generally, lights that flicker five to thirty times per second can trigger a seizure in photosensitive people.

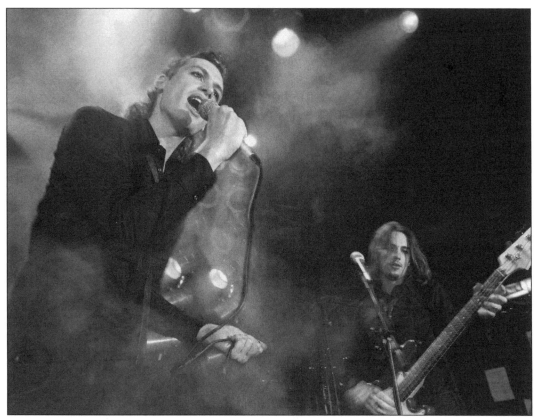

About 3 percent of people with epilepsy are photosensitive; exposure to strobe lights or flashing lights at certain intensities and various visual patterns can trigger seizures.

me but my son's an epileptic,' and they would much rather I suppose naturally talk about success rather than what was certainly perceived as a failure."[5]

Samme Kent, a Floridian, can well remember how, during her teens and early twenties, she and her "adopted" family (people who did not legally adopt but treated her like one of their own) reacted when their son Joseph Woodruff had grand mal seizures. The Woodruffs—Joseph, his older brother, and their parents—lived on three acres in a heavily wooded area in Shady Hills, Florida.

"Joseph was like a brother to me," Samme said, and when he seized "it was a scary thing to watch, it affected all of us—me, his brother and parents, and any friends who were around." Just before an attack, Joseph would "sort of shake his head from side to side and mumble something." Some of Woodruff's friends would "freak out, and others would shy away" when Joseph had a seizure. But "no one made fun of him," and the family or relatives and close friends made sure someone was around to watch over Joseph. After a seizure, "he sometimes slept off and on for three days." Samme explained that she "worried for him" because he would "drive to a job or wherever and did not tell anyone he had epilepsy. Driving through the woods, daylight would flash in and out through the trees, which could trigger a [photogenic] seizure—very risky."[6]

## Accepting the Reality of Epilepsy

Frequently parents say they have difficulty accepting a child's epilepsy diagnosis. In some cases, they don't really want to believe the doctors and are in denial at first. They may seek out support groups to help them deal with the reality.

Parents whose children have seizures need an accurate assessment of their children's potential and to learn how to help them achieve both at home and at school. That, however, does not always happen. Some parents become overprotective and don't allow their children to engage in team sports and other activities. Other parents may feel guilty and believe they somehow caused the disorder. Sometimes parents of epileptic offspring raise them to believe they are unable to accomplish much; as a result, by the time they are teenagers, these young people have low self-esteem. They may become very dependent and have little ambition to succeed.

"The diagnosis of epilepsy, although given to an individual, affects the entire family and its constellation of friendships and other relationships. At onset all are confronted with the immediate need to learn about the disorder and its management. Receiving helpful information and education in the diagnostic phase of a chronic health condition can facilitate coping, because early perceptions may affect long-term adjustment to the condition," says a report by the Institute of Medicine in Washington, DC. The report emphasizes

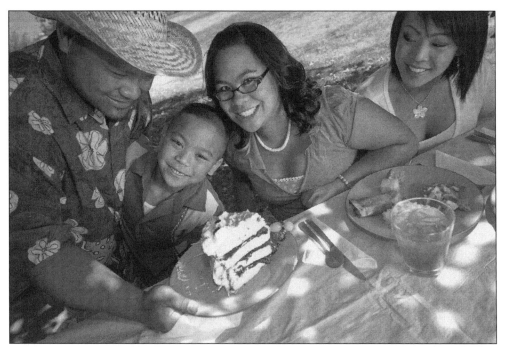

Epilepsy often has a negative impact not only on those with the disorder, but also on families, friends, classmates, coworkers, and others. But most people with epilepsy can enjoy full lives and family activities.

## It Happened to the Boyum Family

Articles about Brett and Heather Boyum's family of Rosemount, Minnesota, and their experiences with epilepsy have appeared online in a variety of forms. In November 2015, for example, journalist Mollie Guthrey reported the family's story, which began in 2002 when the Boyums' son Travis was only four years old. Over several weeks Travis's parents observed that their son would "space out" at times. After consulting with a pediatric neurologist, they learned that Travis had epileptic absence seizures. "We went home that night, and we for sure cried a little bit," Brett told Guthrie. "But then we dug into the research to understand it more. And we decided we weren't going to let epilepsy define his childhood. We refused to let it define him." Travis went on to complete his elementary and high school education, playing football, basketball, and lacrosse.

One night in 2009, Travis's father, Brett Boyum, had a seizure at the age of forty. His wife, Heather, called paramedics, and Brett was treated at a hospital. He was not diagnosed with epilepsy at first, but a year later he had another seizure and learned he had epilepsy and began to take antiseizure medications.[a]

Together the Boyums—Travis, his younger siblings Claire and Tyler, and their parents—are dedicated advocates for epilepsy awareness. Both Travis and his father have been on the board of the Minnesota Epilepsy Foundation, and Heather Boyum is active in epilepsy awareness programs. The family's mission is to serve others affected by seizures through the Minnesota foundation.

Another supporter of the foundation is the courageous University of Minnesota football coach Jerry Kill, who was 2014 Big Ten Coach of the Year. Kill has epilepsy and has had seizures on the football field. He suddenly resigned in November 2015 due to an increase in his seizures, and many of his fans applauded him for being an inspiration for thousands of others with epilepsy. At the time, Travis summed up the situation like this: "I kind of look at it just like football. . . . I mean, you take hits. You have to get a hit, but you have to stand back up and sometimes you get up and you have to go to a different position. I think as a head coach, he [Kill] got knocked down, he will get back up and he will go do something great again."[b] That attitude also applies to Travis himself.

continued educational efforts can play a key role in helping people learn to live with and understand epilepsy and its effects over the life span. Thus, individuals and families need education and skills building throughout the course of the disorder, particularly during times of change, such as an increased frequency of seizures, changes in treatment (e.g., switching medications, starting a new treatment option, discontinuing a medication or other treatment option), and major life transitions (e.g., from youth to adulthood, from adulthood to older adulthood).[7]

## Sudden Unexpected Death in Epilepsy

Families seldom talk or even want to think about sudden unexpected death in epilepsy (SUDEP). It is one of the most frightening aspects of the disorder. SUDEP, as its name implies, happens without warning, often in sleep. Blogger Tom Stanton wrote that SUDEP took his young nephew. "Danny had four seizures that his family knew of, all at night, before the fifth seizure took his life.

Uncontrolled or refractory epilepsy (seizures that resist drug treatment) and habitual tonic clonic seizures at night present two of the greatest risks for SUDEP." After Danny's death, the family set up the Danny Did Foundation to advocate for SUDEP awareness.[8]

Most people with epilepsy live long lives, but an estimated one in one thousand persons die each year from SUDEP. The causes are unknown. Researchers say that some risk factors for SUDEP are frequent tonic-clonic seizures, but they also urge people with epilepsy to discuss with their doctors what their risks might be.

An informative source for information about SUDEP is a pamphlet that appears at http://www.epilepsy.com/sites/core/files/atoms/files/SUDEP_YoungAdults_0.pdf. Another website is sponsored by three organizations, SUDEP Action UK, SUDEP Aware Canada, and Epilepsy Australia. A site that provides information as well as family stories is SUDEP Global Conversation. One account is about Kimberly Laura Bartlett written by her sister Jaimee Bartlett.

Kimberly, who grew up in Massachusetts, died in 2015 due to SUDEP. At the time she was twenty-five years old and "the Operations Manager for . . . a company she started with her dad." She also "was pursuing her Masters in Human Resources Management at Emmanuel College in Boston, Massachusetts," her sister wrote.

## Family Books

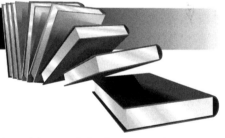

*Living with Epilepsy* by Sara Cohen Christopherson (Abdo Publishing, 2012) is a good read for young people and their families just beginning to learn about epilepsy. The book is addressed to teens and covers basic information about the disorder along with suggestions for readers who have epilepsy. Color photos enhance the book.

A colorful comic book *What's Up with Bill? Medikidz Explain Epilepsy* (Rosen, 2010) is just what the title implies—it explains epilepsy in an entertaining style. Medikidz are a gang of five superheroes from Mediland, which is shaped like a human body. Written by Dr. Kim Chilman-Blair and illustrated by John Taddeo, the comic book is designed to appeal to young teens, but older youth with epilepsy are likely to benefit from the information provided. This comic book is part of a series of Medikidz titles, each dealing with a particular health issue.

In April 2015, Kimberly had a seizure while sleeping. She was rushed to a hospital, and doctors informed her that the seizure was "likely a onetime incident and wouldn't happen again." But on May 11, 2015, Kimberly had another seizure in her sleep and died of SUDEP.

Her death was a major shock to her family and friends. They have established the Living for Kimberly Foundation to spread awareness about epilepsy and Sudden Unexpected Death in Epilepsy.[9]

# THE MILITARY AND EPILEPSY

*"The hectic life triggered me to have my first few seizures which changed my life forever."*
—Andy Nguyen describing his U.S. Army experience[1]

Every year, thousands of young men and women enlist in the U.S. armed services—*if* they meet the requirements, one of which is a high school degree. Many potential enlistees are just out of high school or are dropouts who have passed a GED (General Educational Development test), which is designed for adults over the age of sixteen who have not graduated from high school. Passing the test is equivalent to earning a diploma.

Even if qualified, young people with epilepsy wonder if their disorder will bar them from the military. With all the required physical drills, marches, and sleep deprivation, can they serve in the armed forces? The answer is yes—under certain conditions.

## Some Personal Views

Andy Nguyen has a personal view about his epilepsy and being in the army. He posted his story on CureEpilepsy.org. He describes how seizures were triggered when he was eighteen years old and training for the military. "The hectic life triggered me to have my first few seizures which changed my life forever," he wrote. "Prior to the seizure I had nightmares along with delusional visions of things that weren't there." He noted that epilepsy kept him from serving in the military, and even made him doubt whether he should go on to school because of possible seizures. "Fear holds me back from countless activities but this will be the only life that I'll ever have and I need to experience it all even with a handicap. I encourage everyone who has epilepsy to live their lives to the fullest because even I try everyday with the struggle of worrying that I might die anytime from

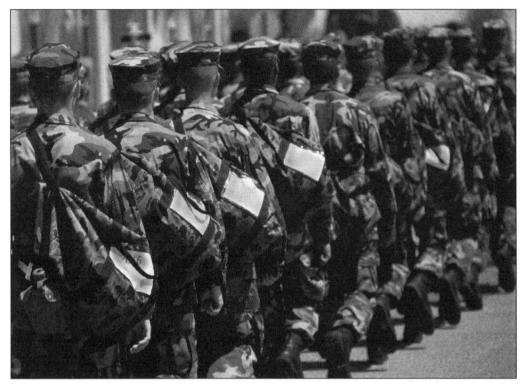

A person with epilepsy can enlist in the army if she or he has been seizure free for at least five years and is not taking antiseizure medication.

a deadly attack." He expressed his hope for a cure, but added, "With or without a cure that can permanitely [*sic*] take away this disease we should all enjoy life and have fun."[2]

In a discussion on ecommunity, comments about failed attempts to join the military underscore how epilepsy changes career plans. For example, one woman wrote: "When I was in high school, I was seizure free for 2 years off medication and I was hoping to join the army after 3 more years (since in order to join you need to be 5 years seizure free off meds). Unfortunately during my senior year I had a terrible seizure. I didn't know about the 5 year rule at this time and when I found out, I was crushed."[3]

## Now You Know

• In the past, any history of seizures after age five prohibited admission into *any* branch of the U.S. armed forces. But the U.S. Department of Defense revised its regulations in 1982, and currently applicants for military service are considered on an individual basis if a person has been seizure-free and without medication for at least five years. The exception is the U.S. Air Force, which generally bars anyone with epilepsy from enlistment. However, the air force accepts recruits who had seizures prior to the age of five as long as a current EEG shows normal results.

The U.S. Department of Defense says in its *Medical Standards for Appointment, Enlistment, or Induction in the Military Services* that "individuals under consideration for appointment, enlistment, or induction into the Military Services" must be

1. Free of contagious diseases that probably will endanger the health of other personnel.
2. Free of medical conditions or physical defects that may require excessive time lost from duty for necessary treatment or hospitalization, or probably will result in separation from the Service for medical unfitness.
3. Medically capable of satisfactorily completing required training.
4. Medically adaptable to the military environment without the necessity of geographical area limitations.
5. Medically capable of performing duties without aggravation of existing physical defects or medical conditions.[a]

If the conditions described are not met, a young person may seek a waiver, and each of the individual armed forces decides whether to grant or deny the waiver. In some cases, a military service will take into account its needs at the time, the specific geographical areas where the person would serve, as well as all information the doctors provide with regard to the impact of the medical condition.

Apart from epilepsy issues in the military, "more than two-thirds of America's young people wouldn't qualify for military service because of physical, behavioral, or educational problems," *Business Insider* reports. "The Pentagon says 71 percent of America's 34 million 17–24 year old population would fail to qualify for enlistment." Although seizures may prevent a person from joining the military or continuing to serve, another problem is obesity. "Major General Allen Batschelet, commander of the U.S. Army Recruiting Command, says obesity is becoming a national security issue." He says that because of obesity, by 2020, "only 2 in 10 would qualify to join the Army."[b]

One twenty-four-year-old posted that he "was diagnosed with epilepsy at age 12," but had been "seizure free for 10 years and was able to join the Air Force in 2011. First thing I did when going to the recruiter is tell him that I had a history of it and he said ok. I had to get my medical record for him and they sent them up through the chain of command and a year and a half later I finally left for basic. . . . The only jobs I am restricted from doing is because of my eye sight and not cause of epilepsy."[4]

## Having Seizures while Serving

A nineteen-year-old in the navy explained on Epilepsy.com that he has had three grand mal seizures since February 2015, and after the first one he was told that he "was dehydrated and to just drink lots of water. About 9 days later after working out I layed [sic] my head down to close my eyes and next thing I knew I was in the hospital, I had one seizure before I made it to the hospital and a worse one in the ER. . . . I was diagnosed with epilepsy and put on medication right away, I was told I'm non-deployable and cannot stay on the ship. . . . I have so many questions as to what my benefits will be because I am told that I will most likely be getting discharged."[5]

On an epilepsy community forum, a twenty-four-year-old navy lieutenant named Phil explained that he was diagnosed with epilepsy after he had several seizures while serving in the Persian Gulf. The first one was "in the middle of the night," he reported, "and my right leg felt 'asleep' and was shaking uncontrollably. The 'asleep' feeling spread to my whole body, and I couldn't move, breathe, or speak. My ears began to 'buzz' very loudly and it felt like I was in another world. An intense pain hit all of my joints and muscles, and then I blacked out."[6]

The navy doctor thought he had "sleep paralysis," but Phil said, "It happened two more times, about once every 4–5 weeks, and on one occasion I lost control of my bladder." During a fourth episode, his roommate witnessed what happened, and as he began to convulse, nearly fell out of his top bunk. "Thankfully, my roommate caught me and laid me on the floor, where I convulsed for about 3–4 minutes. After it was over, he stood me up, and I kept walking into walls and falling down." After half an hour, Phil was finally able to return to his normal behavior, but could not remember what happened. He did not know whether he would be medically discharged or be able to continue his naval career.[7]

Another man serving in the Army National Guard, wrote in 2016 for the community forum: "I recently was diagnosed with a seizure disorder. My seizure types are absence and tonic-clonic (grand mal). I have been suffering with convulsions for about one year with nearly constant migraine headaches on one side. . . . Every time I have gone to drill for the past year, I have had a seizure and lost conscious [*sic*] twice." Nevertheless, in spite of these conditions, he has been unable to get a medical discharge because he explains "the army just keeps pushing my paperwork ever so slowly. They do not want to medically discharge me."[8]

If military members receive a medical discharge they become eligible for monthly compensation and health benefits through the Veterans Administration, which states, "Disability compensation is a monthly benefit paid to Veterans for disabilities resulting from injuries or diseases incurred or aggravated during military service. . . . Generally, Servicemembers who are medically discharged are automatically considered for VA disability compensation."[9]

## Veterans with Epilepsy

Most people who follow the news know that many veterans returning from battle suffer from post-traumatic stress disorder (PTSD)—panic attacks, depression, substance abuse, suicidal thoughts—as well as physical injuries stemming from military combat. There is also much public discussion of traumatic brain injury (TBI) as military men and women return from battles. On the PBS documentary *SEIZED*, a narrator explained, "As far back as World War II, it's been known that half of all soldiers who suffer head wounds in combat will go on to develop epilepsy. Now hundreds of thousands of veterans who fought in Iraq and Afghanistan are coming home with a different kind of damage to their brains—damage they often don't even know they have."[10]

Veterans who have suffered TBI are at risk for epileptic seizures, and U.S. vets deployed since 2001 suffer high rates of epilepsy and other neurological disorders. "The Veterans Health Administration estimates about 100,000 former military service members are seeking treatment for seizures every year, up from 70,000 in 2000," the Tacoma, Washington, *News Tribune* reported. "The rising numbers stem from the traumatic brain injuries that an estimated 20 percent of Iraq and Afghanistan veterans experienced during the wars. Survivors of battlefield explosions often had their heads rattled, fell unconscious and sometimes experienced lasting changes to their memory and moods."[11]

A study by Martin Salinsky, MD, was reported in *Neurology Review* (June 2013), which noted that PTSD "preceded a diagnosis of psychogenic nonepileptic seizures in 58% of military veterans and a diagnosis of epileptic seizures in 14% of military veterans. . . . [Salinsky's] study found that a history of PTSD "was the only significant" factor in predicting "psychogenic seizures in this population."[12]

Yet, epilepsy is seldom associated with veterans, even though the U.S. Veterans Administration (VA) conducted research on epilepsy among veterans during the late 1960s. The VA also set up epilepsy centers such as the Yale Comprehensive Epilepsy Center. "From the mid-1970s through the early 1990s, the VA/

Yale center coordinated the clinical studies of antiepileptic drugs with colleagues in VA medical centers across the United States. These multicenter cooperative studies evolved into the largest controlled trials ever for epilepsy," according to a report from the VA at USMedicine.com. But during the early 1990s, the VA "stepped back from epilepsy research for about 15 years."[13]

## VA Epilepsy Centers

Beginning in the mid-2000s, "major developments in the field changed how researchers understood and physicians treated seizures and epilepsy. . . . In 2008, the VA founded the Epilepsy Centers of Excellence." There are sixteen sites located in cities such as Seattle, Washington; Portland, Oregon; San Francisco, California; Albuquerque, New Mexico; Houston, Texas; Minneapolis, Minnesota; Madison, Wisconsin; Baltimore, Maryland; Miami, Florida; and others. The centers work together to care for veterans with epilepsy.[14]

In February 2016, the VA announced that the epilepsy centers had developed a video series titled *Veterans and Epilepsy: Basic Training.* Stephanie Chen, an epilepsy nurse practitioner with the San Francisco VA Medical Center, explained, "There is a culture of stoicism in the military, which prevents veterans with epilepsy from reaching out to get more information about their epilepsy. Hopefully

### Exceptional Family Member Program (EFMP)

Outside of the military, the EFMP is little known. Members of the armed services are required to enroll in the EFMP if someone in their family—adult or child—has "any physical, emotional, developmental or intellectual disorder that requires special treatment, therapy, education, training, housing or counseling" and "requires any medical care above the level normally provided by a family physician in an outpatient setting," says Carl R. Darnall, Army Medical Center, Fort Hood, Texas. Enrollment is required if military family members have such health conditions as autism, cancer, epilepsy, and other disorders requiring special health care. One of the purposes of the EFMP is "to avoid sending family members to locations that do not have the appropriate medical or educational care."[c]

these videos will show veterans and all individuals living with epilepsy they are not alone."[15]

The videos "address the stigma of epilepsy and educate veterans, their caregivers, and the general public about living with epilepsy. . . . Each video in the series features a veteran sharing his or her personal experiences and unique challenges balancing the medical, personal, and social aspects associated with having recurring seizures." According to the VA, "The goal of the video series is to promote public awareness of the impact of epilepsy in the lives of veterans and to convey that these people are able to live full, productive, successful lives."[16]

# RAISING AWARENESS, SEEKING CURES

*"If we don't have more research for more medications there's going to be a lot
of kids who have run out of options [for epilepsy treatment]"*
—Kathryn Stevens at Teens Speak Up Conference[1]

Many people wonder why there is not already a cure for epilepsy since it has been recognized for millennia. The underlying problem is the variation in causes and types of epilepsy. So scientists have to take many diverse paths as they seek ways to prevent epileptic seizures. They also need funds to pursue research.

Numerous young people with epilepsy have created or sponsored projects to help raise awareness of epilepsy as well as seek donations for research. In 2012, for example, Audrey Kaller, who was diagnosed with epilepsy in her early teens, led a team that raised $35,000 for the Walk to End Epilepsy in Palisades, California. The following year her team raised $50,000, and in 2014 she once again participated in the Palisades walk/run to end epilepsy. She has also traveled to Washington, DC, as an ambassador for Los Angeles Children's Hospital to petition for funds for epilepsy treatment and research.

In May 2016, sixteen-year-old Hannah Enge of Minnesota turned an unfortunate seizure incident into a positive message. The Thief River Falls teenager has had numerous seizures. According to *Fox News*, Hannah has "epileptic, non-epileptic seizures and cataplexy which is described as a strong emotion or laughter that causes a person to suffer sudden physical collapse though remaining conscious."[2]

Hannah suffered a seizure while she was on stage to answer interview questions during a beauty pageant. When she was able to get up, Hannah "explained how her pageant platform, SPARK, played out in front of the whole audience. 'That was one of my many seizures. This is what I've been facing for the last four years. Any change of emotion this is what happens to me. I want to speak for those who can't speak. Those who don't have the opportunity like I have right

## When Is It Okay to Joke?

A sense of humor—being able to joke about having seizures—is a way that some young people who have seizures reduce anxiety and fear among their classmates, friends, and family members. Having a sense of humor about epilepsy is an indication that it is okay to talk about it and thus inform others about seizures. Some people with epilepsy on HealthTalk.org said that "they preferred their good friends to have a laugh about epilepsy rather than take it too seriously or fuss over them." One person noted that seizures can "seem quite scary to talk about, not for me, but for like other people, whereas picturing somebody spontaneously breakdancing out of control is actually quite funny. And that doesn't make it as scary." Still, interviewees on the website made it clear that there is a difference between joking with someone and making jokes about a person. Sometimes humor can be offensive, so it is important to know when and with whom to joke about epilepsy.[a]

here. I ignited my SPARK, thank you,'" Hannah said to the crowd.[3] Her reaction not only showed she had spark, but also a sense of humor.

## Teen Advocates

In 2014, Mayor Ronnie Marks of Athens, Alabama, honored teenager Alexia Lange for her efforts to inform people about epilepsy. Alexia began having multiple epileptic seizures when she was just a year old. When she was two, she had fifty-four seizures in one hour and was in a coma; doctors thought she would not survive. Four times she came near death from seizures. When she was nine years old, she had brain surgery to remove her left frontal lobe. For a year after the surgery she had seizures, but they gradually subsided and stopped suddenly.

As a seventeen-year-old in 2014, Alexia was eager to get involved in epilepsy awareness. She was able to convince Mayor Marks to declare November as Epilepsy Awareness Month. For her part, Alexia has attempted to hand out purple ribbons to symbolize the month. "I just want people to know it's important. . . . Epilepsy is deadly. I'm hoping people can be aware of seizures," she told the Athens *News Courier*.[4]

Another teenager who is an advocate for epilepsy awareness is Craig Mico-lichek of Fond du Lac, Wisconsin. Craig came near death because of seizures while an infant and has intractable epilepsy. He has taken at least nine different medications but they have not controlled his seizures. As a result his memory and cognitive skills have been affected. Craig told a reporter the hardest part of his condition "is the frustration, knowing that I can't do everything I want. . . . Because I know I can do it."[5] In spite of obstacles, Craig, his parents, and older brother Alex are strong advocates for epilepsy awareness.

An additional strong advocate is Kathryn Stevens of Hornell, New York. In April 2016, sixteen-year-old Kathryn attended the annual Teens Speak Up Conference in Washington, DC. She had petit mal when she was in elementary school and then, as she told Hornell's *Evening Tribune*, "I had my first grand mal seizure three years ago on Easter." As her seizures became more frequent and her medications were adjusted, she suffered extreme weight loss and "missed 37 days of school because it was really really bad," she recalled. Stevens also deals with memory loss related to the medications. While at the conference, she spoke to legislators and urged them to fund research for additional antiseizure medica-

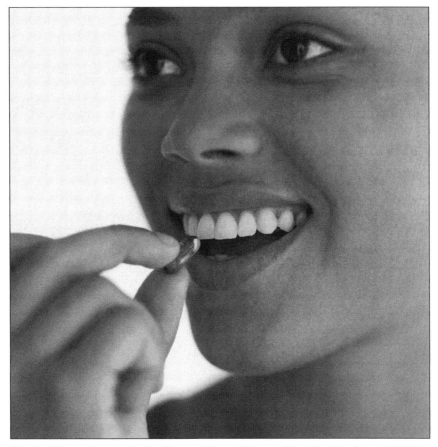

Controlling seizures typically requires taking anti-epileptic drugs (AEDs).

## Purple Day

In 2008, nine-year-old Cassidy Megan of Nova Scotia, Canada, started a Purple Day campaign to increase awareness of epilepsy worldwide. Because of her own experiences with epilepsy, Cassidy wanted to dispel the myths about the disorder. Purple Day is celebrated on March 26, and people from around the globe wear purple to spread the word about epilepsy. In some cities, a "purple man" wears a purple outfit, mask, and hat and cavorts about city streets to heighten epilepsy awareness. Students in many schools across Canada, the United States, Great Britain, and other nations also participate in Purple Day.

tions and "legal access to medical cannabis and cannabis oil." She explained that she was on "the last possible medication for my type of epilepsy. If we don't have more research for more medications there's going to be a lot of kids who have run out of options."[6]

## Advocacy Organizations

The major organization that sponsors walks, marathons, bike rides, and other events for epilepsy awareness is the Epilepsy Foundation in Landover, Maryland, founded in 1968. It has nearly fifty affiliated organizations throughout the United States. The foundation sponsors the National Walk for Epilepsy like the three-mile walk in Washington, DC, in April 2016 which benefited the foundation. The walk was around the Tidal Basin and past the Jefferson Memorial. Another shorter walk was for families, who took a one-mile jaunt around the Washington Monument grounds.

In May 2016, the Epilepsy Foundation launched the new website called Talk-AboutIt.org in partnership with epilepsy advocate and actor Greg Grunberg, whose son had epilepsy in high school. The website raises awareness about seizure symptoms, provides first aid information, and addresses misconceptions about the condition. The foundation announced that numerous celebrities would appear on its website to help educate visitors about epilepsy and seizures. Some of the celebrities include: J. J. Abrams, director of *Star Wars: The Force Awakens*, and

Harrison Ford, *Star Wars* actor; Jennifer Garner of *Alias*; Christopher Gorham of *Covert Affairs*; Chris Pine of *Star Trek*; and Milo Ventimiglia of *Gilmore Girls*.

State affiliates of the Epilepsy Foundation also promote epilepsy education and fund-raisers. Northeast Regional Epilepsy Group is just one group that participates. The group sponsors a Bike-a-Thon to raise awareness and in May 2016, the bike riders traveled through New York's five boroughs (forty miles).[7]

Finding a Cure for Epilepsy and Seizures (FACES) is affiliated with New York University's Langone Medical Center and is directed by renowned neurologist Professor Orrin Devinsky, MD. Langone's FACES has several events each year to seek donations. Its mission "is to improve the quality of life for all those affected by epilepsy and seizures." The organization "funds research to improve epilepsy care, advances new therapies, and fosters a supportive community for children, families and caregivers who live with the challenges of epilepsy."[8]

Many organizations seeking remedies for epilepsy are listed with their addresses and websites at the back of this book. Included is the National Institute of Neurological Disorders and Stroke. NINDS has published a booklet *Hope through Research* with explanations about the type of research being conducted to diminish the effects of epileptic seizures. The publication also describes efforts to identify genes responsible for epileptic conditions, along with helpful information about epilepsy and seizures. The booklet can be accessed online or a published copy can be ordered.[9]

## Advertised "Cures" for Seizures

While there is no evidence that a cure exists for epilepsy aside from surgery, for centuries there have been claims that certain natural products, syrups, gadgets, and specific foods are "cures" for epileptic seizures. Some remedies may help diminish seizures, however, and they include castor oil, garlic, coconut water, Epsom salts, licorice, sesame oil, violet tree flowers, magnesium-rich foods, chamomile tea, oily fish, and various vitamins. Nevertheless, medical experts warn consumers to be cautious about buying vitamin and herbal supplements for epilepsy—so-called natural remedies that are advertised as cures.

"Although vitamins are necessary for good health, large doses of vitamins do not improve the symptoms of epilepsy and may even be harmful," according to WebMD.com. "If necessary, vitamin supplements such as folic acid can help deal with vitamin loss caused by medication. People with epilepsy taking seizure medications do appear to have an increased need for calcium and vitamin D to help keep their bones healthy. . . . Pregnant women also need sufficient folic acid to help prevent birth defects."[10]

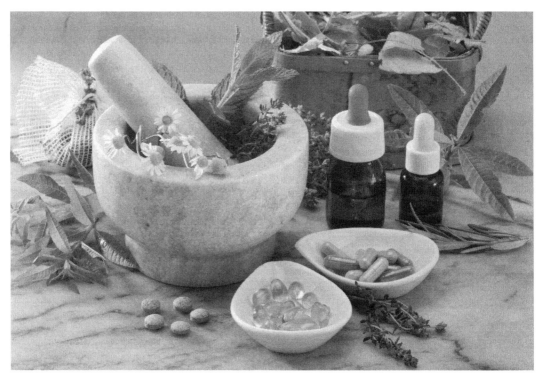

Some claim that certain natural products, tonics, syrups, herbs, and other homeopathic remedies can cure epileptic seizures. ©iStock.com/Pat_Hastings

## Recent Studies and Treatments

NINDS noted in February 1, 2016,

> Scientists are studying the underlying causes of the epilepsies in children, adults, and the elderly, as well as seizures that occur following brain trauma, stroke, and brain tumors. Ongoing research is focused on developing new model systems that can be used to more quickly screen potential new treatments for the epilepsies. The identification of genes or other genetic information that may influence or cause the epilepsies may allow doctors to prevent the disorders or to predict which treatments will be most beneficial to individuals with specific types of epilepsy. Scientists also continue to study how neurotransmitters interact with brain cells to control nerve firing and how non-neuronal cells in the brain contribute to seizures. Researchers funded by the National Institutes of Health have developed a flexible brain implant that could one day be used to treat seizures. Scientists are continually improving MRI and other brain scans that may assist in diagnosing the epilepsies and identify the source, or focus, of the seizures in the brain. Other areas of study include prevention of

seizures and the role of inflammation in epilepsy. Patients may enter trials of experimental drugs and surgical interventions.[11]

As described previously, some epilepsy patients have had brain surgery to stop further seizures. Surgery is an effective option when treatment does not work. The most common type of surgery removes the small area of the brain where seizures originate. Yet, relatively few people who have epilepsy are candidates for surgery and most epileptic patients have to rely on pharmaceuticals (or perhaps cannabis oils) to control their seizures.

In 2013, the U.S. Food and Drug Administration approved NeuroPace, an electronic device known as the responsive neurostimulation system (RNS®), developed in Mountain View, California. Clinical trials have been conducted since it was patented. The NeuroPace is smaller than a playing card and is rounded and looks a bit like a one-dimensional computer mouse. It is surgically implanted under the scalp to help epilepsy patients who do not respond to medication. Two thin wires with electrodes at the end are placed in the brain where seizures originate. The electrodes are designed to detect abnormal brain activity and "zap" it away before it spreads.

One person who has benefited from the NeuroPace is Ian Olsen, who was twenty-seven years old at the time he described his experience. From the time he was eleven, he had had numerous seizures each month—"day or night; awake or asleep." He explained on the website for NeuroPace.com, "As an adolescent I was troubled by the episodes, but didn't know they were seizures and didn't seek help. . . . For years the seizures affected my life. Their onset interrupted me from doing whatever I was doing. They put me and others at risk. . . . They prevented me from driving. They led me to being fired from jobs and limited job options. They caused distress for me and those close to me." After many medications, consultations with several neurologists, and a move from Maryland to California, in 2014 Olsen met Dr. Everett Austin, an epilepsy specialist at Kaiser Hospital in Redwood City. After several consultations, Olsen had the RNS device implanted in February 2015. Over the next few months, he had seizures, but the doctor kept adjusting the timing of the device to prevent attacks from occurring.

Since mid-August 2015, Olsen has not had seizures, and noted, "I can live each day, and complete each task, knowing I won't be inhibited by a seizure. I am more mentally capable. I am able to drive and am less at risk crossing the street, swimming, and standing on high places. I'm more capable of remembering details and performing job responsibilities. Every night I can count on remembering the events of that day." Although he is aware that "different treatments work for different people," in his view everyone who has seizures should know about the RNS device.[12]

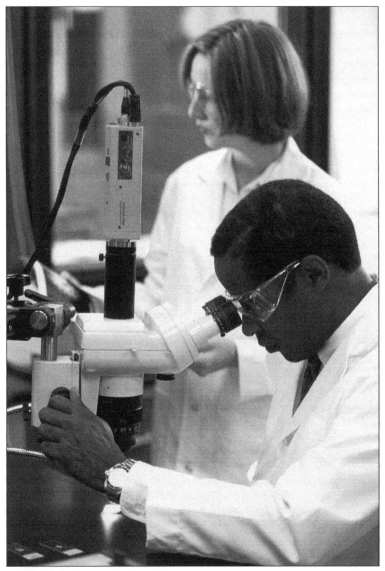

Scientists across the nation and around the world are trying to find cures for epilepsy.

## Continued Research

In spite of the constant need for funds to extend research and develop clinical trials, studies continue. Citizens United for Research in Epilepsy (CURE) noted in its 2013 report that "scientific advances provide renewed hope that a disease modifying therapy or cure is within reach." CURE points to "notable scientific advances" such as greater understanding of how the brain develops, more treatment therapies for epilepsy, and expanded focus on identifying more effective antiseizure drugs.[13]

The U.S. National Library of Medicine reported in April 2016 that a study of the once-a-day drug eslicarbazepine (es-li-car-bazepine) acetate (Aptiom) indicates that it controls seizures as well as other twice-a-day drugs. "The study shows eslicarbazepine to be as effective as the older, more tried-and-true drug, carbamazepine, from which it is derived," said Dr. Sean Hwang, an attending neurologist at Northwell Health's Comprehensive Epilepsy Care Center in Great Neck, New York.[14]

At the University of Florida Health in Gainesville, researchers are studying possible neural cell implants. According to *Space Coast Daily*, researchers have implanted neurons in a mouse model. "Not only did the human stem cells survive after being transplanted, but they also developed into neurons that behave normally within the brain. . . . For people with epilepsy, stem cell transplantation offers the prospect of someday preventing seizures." The report adds, "During the study, implanted human neural stem cells survived for eight weeks in a mouse model and developed into three types of 'connector' neurons called interneurons. . . . With epilepsy, the implanted cells could be used to produce inhibitory neurons to calm the firestorm of overexcited brain cells that cause seizures."[15]

Scientists at Louisiana State University's New Orleans Neuroscience Center of Excellence reported in January 2015 that they had discovered a "novel compound" called Neuroprotectin D-1 that may "curtail the onset and progression of temporal lobe epilepsy." It also "may contribute to the development of anti-epileptic therapies." The researchers "found that brief, small electrical microbursts, or microseizures, occur before the onset of clinical recurrent seizures. When they systemically administered Neuroprotectin D-1 (NPD1), the researchers discovered that NPD1 regulated these bursts of brain electrical activity that not only reduced the aberrant brain cell signaling leading to severe generalized seizures, but also spontaneous recurrent seizures."[16]

In March 2016, MayoClinic.org posted a news release with what appeared to be a riddle: "What do you get when you combine one online contest, two patients, five dogs and 654 data scientists?" The answer: "Hope for patients with epilepsy that their seizures can be reliably predicted, and perhaps prevented."[17]

That hope is based on the results of an online study by the Mayo Clinic, the University of Pennsylvania, and the University of Minnesota, "in which more than 500 teams of data scientists from all over the world analyzed hundreds of hours of recordings of electrical activity in the brains of two people and five dogs before and during epileptic seizures." The lead author, Ben Brickmann, a data scientist at the Mayo Clinic, noted,

Seizure forecasting systems have the potential to help patients with epilepsy lead more normal lives. In order for EEG-based seizure forecasting systems to work effectively, computational algorithms [computer codes/

programs and data] must reliably identify periods of increased probability of seizure occurrence. If these seizure-permissive brain states can be identified, devices designed to warn patients of impending seizures would be possible. Patients could avoid potentially dangerous activities like driving or swimming, and medications could be administered only when needed to prevent impending seizures, reducing overall side effects.[18]

In 2015, the National Institutes of Health awarded a grant to the Mayo Clinic team to continue efforts to develop ways to forecast seizures.

Research in genetics is also being conducted. One study examined DNA samples from sixty-two individuals "who died from SUDEP [sudden unexpected death in epilepsy]" and "nearly one-quarter of them carried mutations linked to cardiac sudden death, suggesting that irregular heart rhythms may play a role in a significant number of deaths in epilepsy. One-quarter also had genetic mutations associated with epilepsy." A "New York University Langone Medical Center study revealed that genetic mutations altering the transmission of electrical impulses in the heart and brain could raise the risk of SUDEP. . . . The study found mutations in 607 genes in brain tissue from patients who died from SUDEP that were not seen in the tissue from the living people."[19]

As researchers continue their efforts to find cures, millions of people worldwide carry on their campaigns to raise awareness of the disorder. An advocacy sign says it plain and simple: "STOP Epilepsy. Spread the Word. It's a No-Brainer!"

# Appendix: EEOC Questions and Answers about Epilepsy

The U.S. Equal Employment Opportunity Commission (EEOC) has posted "Questions & Answers about Epilepsy in the Workplace and the Americans with Disabilities Act (ADA)" on its website. The fifteen-page, single-spaced document explains how the ADA, amended in 2008 (Amendments Act or ADAAA), prohibits discrimination against qualified individuals with disabilities. Even though some people with epilepsy object to being classified as disabled, the ADA contains important legal protections for them in the workplace. The EEOC enforces the employment provisions, and sections of the EEOC document specifically addresses how the ADA applies to job applicants and employees with epilepsy. The document also explains how employers are limited in their ability to ask questions related to epilepsy and to conduct medical examinations at three stages: pre-offer, post-offer, and during employment. The entire document is available on EEOC's website https://www.eeoc.gov/laws/types/epilepsy.cfm.

Part of the Q & A section with *original* formatting follows. But footnotes in the document along with numerous lengthy examples demonstrating various situations have been deleted because of space limits.

OBTAINING, USING, AND DISCLOSING MEDICAL INFORMATION

Title I of the ADA limits an employer's ability to ask questions related to epilepsy and other disabilities and to conduct medical examinations at three stages: pre-offer, post-offer, and during employment.

Job Applicants

*Before an Offer of Employment Is Made*

**1. May an employer ask a job applicant whether she has epilepsy or about her treatment related to epilepsy before making a job offer?**

No. An employer may not ask questions about an applicant's medical condition or require an applicant to have a medical examination before it makes a conditional job offer. This means that an employer *cannot* legally ask an applicant questions such as:

- whether she has epilepsy or seizures;
- whether she uses any prescription drugs; or
- whether she ever has filed for workers' compensation or been injured on a job.

Of course, an employer may ask questions pertaining to the qualifications for, or performance of, the job such as:

- whether an applicant has a driver's license; or
- whether he can operate heavy machinery or equipment.

**2. Does the ADA require an applicant to disclose that she has epilepsy or some other disability before accepting a job offer?**

No. The ADA does not require applicants to voluntarily disclose that they have epilepsy or another disability unless they will need a reasonable accommodation for the application process (for example, permission to bring a service animal to an interview). Some individuals with epilepsy, however, choose to disclose their condition because they want their co-workers or supervisors to know what to do if they have a seizure. Often the decision to disclose depends on the type of seizure a person has, the need for assistance during or after a seizure, the frequency of seizures, and the type of work for which the person is applying.

Sometimes, the decision to disclose depends on whether an individual will need a reasonable accommodation to perform the job (for example, breaks to take medication). A person with epilepsy, however, may request an accommodation after becoming an employee even if she did not do so when applying for the job or after receiving the job offer.

**3. May an employer ask any follow-up questions if an applicant voluntarily reveals that she has epilepsy?**

No. An employer generally may not ask an applicant who has voluntarily disclosed that she has epilepsy any questions about her epilepsy, its treatment, or its prognosis. However, if an applicant voluntarily discloses that she **has epilepsy and the employer reasonably believes that she will require an accommodation to perform the job because of her epilepsy or treatment**, the employer may ask whether the applicant will need an accommodation and what type. The employer must keep any information an applicant discloses about her medical condition confidential. (*See* "Keeping Medical Information Confidential.")

*After an Offer of Employment Is Made*

After making a job offer, an employer may ask questions about the applicant's health (including questions about the applicant's disability) and may require a medical examination, as long as all applicants for the same type of job are treated equally (that is, all applicants are asked the same questions and are required to take the same examination). After an employer has obtained basic medical information from all individuals who have received job offers, it may ask specific individuals for more medical information if it is medically related to the previously obtained medical information. For example, if an employer asks all applicants post-offer about their general physical and mental health, it can ask individuals who disclose a particular illness, disease, or impairment for more medical information or require them to have a medical examination related to the condition disclosed.

**4. What may an employer do when it learns that an applicant has epilepsy after he has been offered a job but before he starts working?**

When an applicant discloses after he has received a conditional job offer that he has epilepsy, an employer may ask the applicant additional questions about his epilepsy, such as whether he has held the same or a similar job since his diagnosis; whether he takes any medication; whether he still has seizures and, if so, what type; how long it takes him to recover after a seizure; and/or, whether he will need assistance if he has a seizure at work. The employer also may send the applicant for a follow-up medical examination or ask him to submit documentation from his doctor answering questions specifically designed to assess the applicant's ability to perform the job's functions safely. Permissible follow-up questions at this stage differ from those at the pre-offer stage when an employer only may ask an applicant who voluntarily discloses a disability whether she needs an accommodation to perform the job and what type.

An employer may not withdraw an offer from an applicant with epilepsy if the applicant is able to perform the essential functions of the job, with or without reasonable accommodation, without posing a direct threat (that is, a significant risk of substantial harm) to the health or safety of herself or others that cannot be eliminated or reduced through reasonable accommodation. ("Reasonable accommodation" is discussed in Questions 10 through 15. "Direct threat" is discussed in Questions 6 and 16 through 19.)

Employees

The ADA strictly limits the circumstances under which an employer may ask questions about an employee's medical condition or require the employee to have a medical examination. Once an employee is on the job, his actual performance is the best measure of ability to do the job.

**5. When may an employer ask an employee whether epilepsy, or some other medical condition, may be causing her performance problems?**

Generally, an employer may ask disability-related questions or require an employee to have a medical examination when it knows about a particular employee's medical condition, has observed performance problems, and reasonably believes that the problems are related to the medical condition. At other times, an employer may ask for medical information when it has observed symptoms, such as extreme fatigue or irritability, or has received reliable information from someone else (for example, a family member or co-worker) indicating that the employee may have a medical condition that is causing performance problems. Often, however, poor job performance is unrelated to a medical condition and generally should be handled in accordance with an employer's existing policies concerning performance.

**6. May an employer require an employee on leave because of epilepsy to provide documentation or have a medical examination before allowing her to return to work?**

Yes. If the employer has a reasonable belief that the employee may be unable to perform her job or may pose a direct threat to herself or others, the employer may ask for medical information. However, the employer may obtain only the information needed to make an assessment of the employee's *present* ability to perform her job and to do so safely.

**7. Are there any other instances when an employer may ask an employee with epilepsy about her condition?**

Yes. An employer also may ask an employee about epilepsy when it has a reasonable belief that the employee will be unable to safely perform the essential functions of her job because of epilepsy. In addition, an employer may ask an employee about her epilepsy to the extent the information is necessary:

- to support the employee's request for a reasonable accommodation needed because of her epilepsy;
- to verify the employee's use of sick leave related to her epilepsy if the employer requires all employees to submit a doctor's note to justify their use of sick leave; or
- to enable the employee to participate in a voluntary wellness program.

Keeping Medical Information Confidential

With limited exceptions, an employer must keep confidential any medical information it learns about an applicant or employee. Under the following circumstances, however, an employer may disclose that an employee has epilepsy:

- to supervisors and managers in order to provide a reasonable accommodation or to meet an employee's work restrictions;
- to first aid and safety personnel if an employee would need emergency treatment or require some other assistance if she had a seizure at work;
- to individuals investigating compliance with the ADA and similar state and local laws; and
- where needed for workers' compensation or insurance purposes (for example, to process a claim).

**8. May an employer tell employees who ask why their co-worker is allowed to do something that generally is not permitted (such as have more breaks) that she is receiving a reasonable accommodation?**

No. Telling co-workers that an employee is receiving a reasonable accommodation amounts to a disclosure that the employee has a disability. Rather than disclosing that the employee is receiving a reasonable accommodation, the employer should focus on the importance of maintaining the privacy of all employees and emphasize that its policy is to refrain from discussing the work situation of any employee with co-workers. Employers may be able to avoid many of these kinds of questions by training all employees on the requirements of equal employment opportunity laws, including the ADA.

Additionally, an employer will benefit from providing information about reasonable accommodations to all of its employees. This can be done in a number of ways, such as through written reasonable accommodation procedures, employee handbooks, staff meetings, and periodic training. This kind of proactive approach may lead to fewer questions from employees who misperceive co-worker accommodations as "special treatment."

**9. If an employee has a seizure at work, may an employer explain to other employees or managers that the employee has epilepsy?**

No. Although the employee's co-workers and others in the workplace who witness the seizure naturally may be concerned, an employer may not reveal that the employee has epilepsy. Rather, the employer should assure everyone present that the situation is under control. The employer also should follow the employee's plan of action if one has been created.

An employee may voluntarily choose to tell her co-workers and others that she has epilepsy and provide them with helpful information, such as how to recognize when she is having a seizure, how long her seizures generally last, what, if anything, should be done if she has a seizure, and how long it generally takes her to recover. However, even when an employee voluntarily discloses that she has epilepsy, the employer must keep this information confidential consistent with the ADA. An employer also may not explain to other employees why an employee with epilepsy has been absent from work if the absence is related to her epilepsy or another disability.

ACCOMMODATING EMPLOYEES WITH EPILEPSY

The ADA requires employers to provide adjustments or modifications—called reasonable accommodations—to enable applicants and employees with disabilities to enjoy equal employment opportunities unless doing so would be an undue hardship (that is, a significant difficulty or expense). Accommodations vary depending on the needs of the individual with a disability. Not all employees with epilepsy will need an accommodation or require the same accommodations, and most of the accommodations a person with epilepsy might need will involve little or no cost. An employer must provide a reasonable accommodation that is needed because of the epilepsy itself, the effects of medication, or both. For example, an employer may have to accommodate an employee who is unable to work while undergoing diagnostic tests to determine the reason for her seizures or because of the side effects of medication. An employer, however, has no obligation to monitor an employee's medical treatment or to make sure she is getting enough rest or taking medication as prescribed.

**10. What other types of reasonable accommodations may employees with epilepsy need?**

Some employees may need one or more of the following accommodations:

- breaks to take medication
- leave to seek or recuperate from treatment or adjust to medication
- a private area to rest after having a seizure
- a rubber mat or carpet to cushion a fall
- adjustments to a work schedule

Although these are some examples of the types of accommodations commonly requested by employees with epilepsy, other employees may need different changes or adjustments. Employers should ask the particular employee requesting an accommodation what she needs that will help her do her job. There also are extensive public and private resources to help employers identify reasonable accommodations. For example, the website for the Job Accommodation Network (JAN) (www. askjan. org/media/epilepsy. html) provides information about many types of accommodations for employees with epilepsy.

### 11. How does an employee with epilepsy request a reasonable accommodation?

There are no "magic words" that a person has to use when requesting a reasonable accommodation. A person simply has to tell the employer that she needs an adjustment or change at work because of her epilepsy. A request for reasonable accommodation also can come from a family member, friend, health professional, or other representative on behalf of a person with epilepsy.

### 12. May an employer request documentation when an employee who has epilepsy requests a reasonable accommodation?

Yes. An employer may request reasonable documentation where a disability or the need for reasonable accommodation is not known or obvious. An employer, however, is entitled only to documentation sufficient to establish that the employee has epilepsy and to explain why an accommodation is needed. A request for an employee's entire medical record, for example, would be inappropriate as it likely would include information about conditions other than the employee's epilepsy.

### 13. Does an employer have to grant every request for a reasonable accommodation?

No. An employer does not have to provide an accommodation if doing so will be an undue hardship. Undue hardship means that providing the reasonable accommodation would result in significant difficulty or expense. An employer also does not have to eliminate an essential function of a job as a reasonable accommodation, tolerate performance that does not meet its standards, or excuse violations of conduct rules that are job-related and consistent with business necessity and that the employer applies consistently to all employees (such as rules prohibiting violence, threatening behavior, theft, or destruction of property).

If more than one accommodation would be effective, the employee's preference should be given primary consideration, although the employer is not required to provide the employee's first choice of reasonable accommodation. If a requested accommodation is too difficult or expensive, an employer may choose to provide an easier or less costly accommodation as long as it is effective in meeting the employee's needs.

**14. May an employer be required to provide more than one accommodation for the same employee with epilepsy?**

Yes. The duty to provide a reasonable accommodation is an ongoing one. Although some employees with epilepsy may require only one reasonable accommodation, others may need more than one. For example, an employee with epilepsy may require leave because of frequent seizures and later may request a part-time or modified schedule to get more rest to control her seizures. An employer must consider each request for a reasonable accommodation and determine whether it would be effective and whether providing it would pose an undue hardship.

**15. May an employer automatically deny a request for leave from someone with epilepsy because the employee cannot specify an exact date of return?**

No. Granting leave to an employee who is unable to provide a fixed date of return may be a reasonable accommodation. Although epilepsy often can be successfully controlled, some individuals may be need to take extended leave because of the frequency or severity of their seizures and may be able to provide only an *approximate* date of return (for example, "in six to eight weeks," "in about three months"). In such situations, or in situations in which a return date must be postponed because of unforeseen medical developments, employees should stay in regular communication with their employers to inform them of their progress and discuss the need for continued leave beyond what originally was granted. The employer also has the right to require that the employee provide periodic updates on his condition and possible date of return. After receiving these updates, the employer may reevaluate whether continued leave constitutes an undue hardship.

**16. If an employee does not have a driver's license because of epilepsy, does an employer have to eliminate driving from his job duties?**

It depends. If driving is an essential function of a job, an employer does not have to eliminate it. However, an employer should carefully consider whether driving actually is an essential job function, a marginal job function, or simply one way of accomplishing an essential function. If an accommodation is available that would enable an employee with epilepsy to perform a function that most employees would perform by driving, then the employer must provide the accommodation, absent undue hardship. Similarly, if driving is a marginal (or non-essential) function, the fact that an individual with epilepsy does not have a driver's license cannot be used to deny the individual an employment opportunity.

CONCERNS ABOUT SAFETY

When it comes to safety, an employer should be careful not to act on the basis of myths, fears, generalizations, or stereotypes about epilepsy. Instead, the employer should evaluate each individual on his knowledge, skills, experience, and how having epilepsy affects him.

**17. When may an employer refuse to hire, terminate, or temporarily restrict the duties of a person with epilepsy because of safety concerns?**

An employer only may exclude an individual with epilepsy from a job for safety reasons when the individual poses a direct threat. A "direct threat" is a significant risk of substantial harm to the individual or others that cannot be eliminated or reduced through reasonable accommodation. This determination must be based on objective, factual evidence, including the best recent medical evidence and advances in the treatment of epilepsy.

In making a direct threat assessment, the employer must evaluate the individual's present ability to safely perform the job. The employer also must consider:

1. the duration of the risk;
2. the nature and severity of the potential harm;
3. the likelihood that the potential harm will occur; and
4. the imminence of the potential harm.

The harm must be serious and likely to occur, not remote or speculative. Finally, the employer must determine whether any reasonable accommodation (for example, temporarily limiting an employee's duties, temporarily reassigning an employee, or placing an employee on leave) would reduce or eliminate the risk.

**18. May an employer require an employee who has had a seizure at work to submit periodic notes from his doctor indicating that his epilepsy is under control?**

Yes, but only if the employer has a reasonable belief that the employee will pose a direct threat if he does not regularly see his doctor. In determining whether to require periodic documentation, the employer should consider the safety risks associated with the position the employee holds, the consequences of the employee's inability or impaired ability to perform his job, how long the employee has had epilepsy, and how many seizures the employee has had on the job.

**19. What should an employer do when another federal law prohibits it from hiring anyone who has epilepsy?**

If a federal law prohibits an employer from hiring a person with epilepsy, the employer is not liable under the ADA. The employer should be certain, however, that compliance with the law actually is required, not voluntary. The employer also should be sure that the law does not contain any exceptions or waivers. For example, although the regulations of the U.S. Department of Transportation's Federal Motor Carrier Safety Administration (FMCSA) provide that a person is qualified to drive a commercial motor vehicle if he has no established medical history or clinical diagnosis of epilepsy or any other condition which is likely to cause loss of consciousness or any loss of ability to control a commercial motor vehicle, an individual with epilepsy may apply for an exemption where he can show that safety would not be diminished by granting the exemption.

HARASSMENT

The ADA prohibits harassment, or offensive conduct, based on disability just as other federal laws prohibit harassment based on race, sex, color, national origin, religion, age, and genetic information. Offensive conduct may include, but is not limited to, offensive jokes, slurs, epithets or name calling, physical assaults or threats, intimidation, ridicule or mockery, insults or put-downs, offensive objects or pictures, and interference with work performance. Although the law does not prohibit simple teasing, offhand comments, or isolated incidents that are not very serious, harassment is illegal when it is so frequent or severe that it creates a hostile or offensive work environment or when it results in an adverse employment decision (such as the victim being fired or demoted).

## 20. What should employers do to prevent and correct harassment?

Employers should make clear that they will not tolerate harassment based on disability or on any other basis. This can be done in a number of ways, such as through a written policy, employee handbooks, staff meetings, and periodic training. The employer should emphasize that harassment is prohibited and that employees should promptly report such conduct to a manager. Finally, the employer should immediately conduct a thorough investigation of any report of harassment and take swift and appropriate corrective action. For more information on the standards governing harassment under all of the EEO laws, see www.eeoc.gov/policy/docs/harassment.html.

## RETALIATION

The ADA prohibits retaliation by an employer against someone who opposes discriminatory employment practices, files a charge of employment discrimination, or testifies or participates in any way in an investigation, proceeding, or litigation related to a charge of employment discrimination. It is also unlawful for an employer to retaliate against someone for requesting a reasonable accommodation. Persons who believe that they have experienced retaliation may file a charge of retaliation with the EEOC as described below.

## HOW TO FILE A CHARGE OF EMPLOYMENT DISCRIMINATION

Against Private Employers and State/Local Governments

Any person who believes that his or her employment rights have been violated on the basis of disability and wants to make a claim against an employer must file a charge of discrimination with the EEOC. A third party may also file a charge on behalf of another person who believes that he or she experienced discrimination. . For example, a family member, social worker, or other representative can file a charge on behalf of someone who is incapacitated because of epilepsy. The charge must be filed by mail or in person with the local EEOC office within 180 days from the date of the alleged violation. The 180-day filing deadline is extended to 300 days if a state or local anti-discrimination agency has the authority to grant or seek relief as to the challenged unlawful employment practice.

The EEOC will send the parties a copy of the charge and may ask for responses and supporting information. Before formal investigation, the EEOC may select the charge for EEOC's mediation program. Both parties have to agree to mediation, which may prevent a time-consuming investigation of the charge. Participation in mediation is free, voluntary, and confidential.

If mediation is unsuccessful, the EEOC investigates the charge to determine if there is "reasonable cause" to believe discrimination has occurred. If reasonable cause is found, the EEOC will then try to resolve the charge with the employer. In some cases, where the charge cannot be resolved, the EEOC will file a court action. If the EEOC finds no discrimination, or if an attempt to resolve the charge fails and the EEOC decides not to file suit, it will issue a notice of a "right to sue," which gives the charging party 90 days to file a court action. A charging party can also request a notice of a "right to sue" from the EEOC 180 days after the charge was first filed with the Commission, and may then bring suit within 90 days after receiving the notice. For a detailed description of the process, you can visit our website at www.eeoc.gov/employees/howtofile.cfm.

Against the Federal Government

If you are a federal employee or job applicant and you believe that a federal agency has discriminated against you, you have a right to file a complaint. Each agency is required to post information about how to contact the agency's EEO Office. You can contact an EEO Counselor by calling the office responsible for the agency's EEO complaints program. Generally, you must contact the EEO Counselor within 45 days from the day the discrimination occurred. In most cases the EEO Counselor will give you the choice of participating either in EEO counseling or in an alternative dispute resolution (ADR) program, such as a mediation program.

If you do not settle the dispute during counseling or through ADR, you can file a formal discrimination complaint against the agency with the agency's EEO Office. You must file within 15 days from the day you receive notice from your EEO Counselor about how to file. Once you have filed a formal complaint, the agency will review the complaint and decide whether or not the case should be dismissed for a procedural reason (for example, your claim was filed too late). If the agency doesn't dismiss the complaint, it will conduct an investigation. The agency has 180 days from the day you filed your complaint to finish the investigation. When the investigation is finished, the agency will issue a notice giving you two choices: either request a hearing before an EEOC Administrative Judge or ask the agency to issue a decision as to whether the discrimination occurred. For a detailed description of the process, you can visit our website at www.eeoc.gov/federal/fed_employees/complaint_overview.cfm.

# Notes

## Chapter 1

1. Kayla Brown, "My WebMD: A Teen Copes with Epilepsy," reviewed by Brunilda Nazario, WebMD.com, n.d., http://www.webmd.com/epilepsy/features/teen-copes-with-epilepsy (accessed June 12, 2016).
2. See Epilepsy Foundation, "Epilepsy Statistics," Epilepsy.com, n.d., http://www.epilepsy.com/learn/epilepsy-statistics (accessed April 28, 2016).
3. See "Epilepsy Facts," CureEpilepsy.org, n.d., http://www.cureepilepsy.org/aboutepilepsy/facts.asp (accessed April 29, 2016).
4. Angel Princess Maria, "Not Feeling Wanted Places," Epilepsy Foundation, Teen Zone, February 28, 2016, http://epilepsyfoundation.ning.com/forum/topics/not-feeling-wanted-places (accessed April 26, 2016).
5. "Don't Freak Out about Epilepsy," YouTube video, posted by pscribner, December 1, 2006, https://www.youtube.com/watch?v=2ey67zwLxok&noredirect=1 (accessed April 28, 2016).
6. Brown, "My WebMD: A Teen Copes with Epilepsy."
7. See "Seizures," MedlinePlus, n.d., https://www.nlm.nih.gov/medlineplus/seizures.html (accessed May 1, 2016).
8. "Epilepsy," reviewed by Harry S. Abram, MD, KidsHealth.org, June 2013, http://kidshealth.org/en/teens/epilepsy.html# (accessed April 28, 2016).
9. See "Types of Seizures," EFEPA.org, n.d., www.efepa.org/living-with-epilepsy/types-of-seizures/ (accessed June 5, 2016).
10. See "Brain Basics: Know Your Brain," NIH.gov, n.d., http://www.ninds.nih.gov/disorders/brain_basics/know_your_brain.htm (accessed July 19, 2016).
11. Phylis Feiner Johnson, "Conditions Commonly Misdiagnosed as Epilepsy," EpilepsyTalk.com, February 17, 2010, https://epilepsytalk.com/2010/02/17/conditions-commonly-misdiagnosed-as-epilepsy/ (accessed June 5, 2016).
12. S. Marc Testa, Gregory L. Krauss, Ronald P. Lesser, and Jason Brandt, "Stressful Life Event Appraisal and Coping in Patients with Psychogenic Seizures and Those with Epilepsy," *Seizure*, February 11, 2012, http://www.seizure-journal.com/article/S1059-1311(12)00033-7/pdf (accessed June 13, 2016).
13. Epilepsy Foundation, "The Truth about Psychogenic NonEpileptic Seizures," Epilepsy.com, n.d., http://www.epilepsy.com/article/2014/3/truth-about-psychogenic-nonepileptic-seizures (accessed June 6, 2016).
14. Sheena Jones, "Radio Legend Garrison Keillor Suffers Second Seizure," CNN.com, updated June 4, 2016, http://www.cnn.com/2016/06/03/health/garrison-keillor-brain-seizure/ (accessed June 5, 2016).
15. Jennifer Warner, "Seizures in Vets Often Misdiagnosed," reviewed by Laura J. Martin, MD, WebMD.com, September 6, 2011, http://www.webmd.com/mental-health/news/20110906/cause-of-seizures-in-vets-hard-to-pinpoint (accessed June 6, 2016).

a. John R. Hughes, "Did All Those Famous People Have Epilepsy," UTSouthwestern.edu, November 11, 2004, http://www4.utsouthwestern.edu/swneurosurg/Did_all_those_famous_people_really_have_epilepsy.pdf (accessed May 1, 2016).

b. See "Brain Basics: Know Your Brain," NIH.gov, n.d., http://www.ninds.nih.gov/disorders/brain_basics/know_your_brain.htm (accessed July 19, 2016).

## Chapter 2

1. Anonymous, "Living with Epilepsy Stigma," GirlswithNerve.com, June 17, 2015, http://girlswithnerve.com/living-with-epilepsy-stigma/ (accessed June 15, 2016).

2. See "Room 3: Diagnosis," Epilepsie Museum, n.d., http://www.epilepsiemuseum.de/alt/body_diagnostiken.html (accessed May 1, 2016).

3. See "History of the Minnesota School for Feeble-Minded and Colony for Epileptics," MN.gov, n.d., http://mn.gov/mnddc/past/pdf/10s/10/10-HMS-UNK.pdf (accessed June 4, 2016).

4. Lori Jane Gliha, "Forced Sterilization Nurse: 'I Can See Now That It Was So Wrong,'" *Flagship Blog*, March 24, 2014, http://america.aljazeera.com/watch/shows/america-tonight/america-tonight-blog/2014/3/24/forced-sterilizationnurseicanseenowthatitwassowrong.html (accessed May 15, 2016).

5. George K. York III and David A. Steinberg, "Hughlings Jackson's Neurological Ideas," *Brain: A Journal of Neurology*, revised July 31, 2011, accepted August 3, 2011, http://brain.oxfordjournals.org/content/134/10/3106.explore (accessed May 1, 2016).

6. Epilepsy Foundation, "When Epilepsy Goes By Another Name," epilepsy.com, March 2014, http://www.epilepsy.com/article/2014/3/when-epilepsy-goes-another-name (accessed July 15, 2016).

7. A. Awaritefe, A. C. Longe, and M. Awaritefe, "Epilepsy and Psychosis: A Comparison of Societal Attitudes," *Epilepsia*, January–February 1985, http://www.ncbi.nlm.nih.gov/pubmed/3971944?dopt=Abstract (accessed July 16, 2016).

8. Jerrold E. Levy, Raymond Neutra, and Dennis Parker, *Hand Trembling, Frenzy Witchcraft, and Moth Madness: A Study of Navajo Seizure Disorders* (Tucson: University of Arizona Press, 1995 paperback edition), p. 41.

9. "Award-Winning Actor Danny Glover Featured on 'Sharing Miracles,'" PRNewswire.com, October 23, 2009, http://www.prnewswire.com/news-releases/award-winning-actor-danny-glover-featured-on-sharing-miracles-65774847.html (accessed May 1, 2016).

a. See "Epilepsy 'Cures,'" CenterforInquiry.net, February 24, 2015, www.centerforinquiry.net/blogs/entry/epilepsy_cures/ (accessed May 28, 2016); also see "He Cures Fits," James Joyce Online Notes, http://www.jjon.org/joyce-s-environs/root (accessed June 8, 2016).

## Chapter 3

1. Rachel, "Rachel's Story: I Am Not Alone Anymore," LivingWellwithEpilepsy.com, April 2016, http://livingwellwithepilepsy.com/category/personal-epilepsy-stories (accessed June 15, 2016).

2. Emily, "Emily's Perspective: On Auras," LivingWellwithEpilepsy.com, April 29, 2016, http://livingwellwithepilepsy.com/category/emilys-perspective (accessed May 3, 2016).

3. Kathlyn Gay and Sean McGarrahan, *Epilepsy: The Ultimate Teen Guide* (Lanham, MD: Scarecrow Press, 2002), pp. 20–22.

4. Gay and McGarrahan, *Epilepsy*, pp. 33–34.

5. Barbara Buoy, "This Is My Story," Epilepsy.com, February 22, 2016, http://www.epilepsy.com/article/2016/2/my-story-barbra-buoy (accessed April 23, 2016).

6. Carmen McCollum, "Lake Station Teen Tackles Epilepsy by Raising Awareness," NWI.com, October 5, 2015, http://www.nwitimes.com/news/local/lake-station-teen-tackles-epilepsy-by-raising-awarness/article_54718e6c-6f95-5aec-b4fa-29ad951d6129.html (accessed July 18, 2016).

7. Sophie Punke, "Sophie's Story: A Teen Experience with Seizures," LivingWellwithEpilepsy.com, August 30, 2013, http://livingwellwithepilepsy.com/2013/personal-epilepsy-stories/sophies-story-teen-experience.html (accessed May 3, 2016).

8. Layna, "Layna & Epilepsy," CureEpilepsy.org, n.d., http://www.cureepilepsy.org/share/my-story.asp?story=10 (accessed January 13, 2016).

a. Ernest Ward, DVM, "Seizures—General for Dogs," VCAHospitals.com, n.d., http://www.vcahospitals.com/main/pet-health-information/article/animal-health/seizures-general-for-dogs/903 (accessed June 10, 2016).

# Chapter 4

1. Monique, "Monique's Story," LivingWellwithEpilepsy.com, June 2016, http://livingwellwithepilepsy.com/2016/blog-relay/jun-16-lwwe-posts/epilepsy-and-my-career-goals.html (accessed June 15, 2016).

2. See "Chandler Jahnke," EpilepsyChicago.org, n.d., http://www.epilepsychicago.org/wp-content/uploads/2015/04/Chandler-face.pdf (accessed May 30, 2016).

3. See "A Closer Look at MRI," EpilepsySociety.org, n.d., https://www.epilepsysociety.org.uk/closer-look-mri#.VyooUuRvwdU (accessed May 4, 2016).

4. Celeste E. Whittaker, "Parents: Let Our Teen Take Medical Marijuana," *Courier-Post*, June 16, 2015, http://www.courierpostonline.com/story/news/local/south-jersey/2015/06/16/maple-shade-parents-suing-medical-marijuana/28804985/ (accessed June 12, 2016).

5. Whittaker, "Parents."

6. Susan K. Livio, "N.J. School 1st in Nation to Allow Medical Marijuana for Students," NJ.com, November 12, 2015, http://www.nj.com/politics/index.ssf/2015/11/nj_teens_school_adopts_medical_marijuana_policy_to.html (accessed June 12, 2016).

7. Sanjay Gupta, "Dr. Sanjay Gupta: It's Time for a Medical Marijuana Revolution," CNN.com, updated April 20, 2015, http://www.cnn.com/2015/04/16/opinions/medical-marijuana-revolution-sanjay-gupta/ (accessed July 1, 2015).

8. Saundra Young, "Marijuana Stops Child's Severe Seizures," CNN.com, August 7, 2013, http://www.cnn.com/2013/08/07/health/charlotte-child-medical-marijuana/ (accessed July 3, 2015).

9. Adam Howard, "Senators Unveil Groundbreaking, Bipartisan Medical Marijuana Bill," MSNBC.com, March 10, 2015, http://www.msnbc.com/msnbc/senators-unveil-groundbreaking-birpartisan-medical-marijuana-bill (accessed May 6, 2016).

10. See "25 Legal Medical Marijuana States and DC," ProCon.org, last updated June 28, 2016, http://medicalmarijuana.procon.org/view.resource.php?resourceID=000881 (accessed August 19, 2016).
11. See "Seizure Diary," EpilepsySociety.org, n.d., https://www.epilepsysociety.org.uk/sites/default/files/attachments/SeizurediaryA4versionJuly2015.pdf (accessed May 12, 2016).
12. See "Epilepsy Foundation My Seizure Diary," Epilepsy.com, n.d., http://www.epilepsy.com/get-help/my-epilepsy-diary (accessed May 12, 2016).

a. Kristen Aaron, "Rare Tour of the Only Federal Weed Farm in America," CNN.com, April 20, 2015, http://www.cnn.com/2015/04/17/health/weed-farm-tour/ (accessed May 5, 2016).
b. Alex Rogers, "Uncle Sam Will Buy $69 Million Worth of Pot from Ole Miss," *Time*, March 23, 2015, http://time.com/3755253/university-mississippi-marijuana/ (accessed May 5, 2016).

# Chapter 5

1. "Epilepsy Laser Surgery Gives Teen Normal Life" (news release), ClevelandClinic.org, April 21, 2016, https://newsroom.clevelandclinic.org/2016/04/21/epilepsy-laser-surgery-gives-teen-normal-life/ (accessed September 20, 2016).
2. Howard L. Weiner, MD, and Joseph I. Sirven, MD, "Surgery," Epilepsy.com, reviewed August 2013, http://www.epilepsy.com/learn/treating-seizures-and-epilepsy/surgery (accessed May 8, 2016).
3. Neil Lava, MD, "Epilepsy: Surgical Options for Epilepsy, WebMD.com, July 20, 2014, http://www.webmd.com/epilepsy/surgical-options-epilepsy?page=2 (accessed May 8, 2016).
4. Segann March, "16-Year-Old Boy Gets a Holiday Miracle," *Shreveport Times*, December 23, 2015, http://www.shreveporttimes.com/story/news/2015/12/23/16-year-old-boy-gets-holiday-miracle/77748422/ (accessed May 8, 2016).
5. Nick Lawton, "Logansport Teen Receives New Surgery to Eliminate Epileptic Seizures," KSLA.com, December 22, 2015, http://www.ksla.com/story/30814928/logansport-teen-receives-new-surgery-to-eliminate-epileptic-seizures (accessed May 7, 2016).
6. Charles Pannunzio, "Manhattan Beach Teen Cured of Epilepsy, Works to Bring Trojans, Bruins Together," *Daily Breeze*, November 15, 2016, http://www.dailybreeze.com/health/20141115/manhattan-beach-teen-cured-of-epilepsy-works-to-bring-trojans-bruins-together (accessed June 7, 2016).
7. Susan Pietsch-Escueta, "Los Altos High School Presents the Courage Award to Angel Ojeda, a Teen with Epilepsy and a 'Teen Speak-Up' Advocate," EndEpilepsy.org, May 13, 2016, http://endepilepsy.org/los-altos-high-school-presents-the-courage-award-to-angel-ojeda-a-teen-with-epilepsy-and-a-teen-speak-up-advocate/ (accessed June 2, 2016).
8. Media Library, "Epilepsy Laser Surgery Gives Teen Normal Life," ClevelandClinic.org, April 21, 2016, https://newsroom.clevelandclinic.org/2016/04/21/epilepsy-laser-surgery-gives-teen-normal-life/ (accessed May 7, 2016).
9. Media Library, "Epilepsy Laser Surgery."
10. Mayo Clinic staff, "Vagus Nerve Stimulation," MayoClinic.org, n.d., http://www.mayoclinic.org/tests-procedures/vagus-nerve-stimulation/home/ovc-20167755 (accessed May 7, 2016).
11. Sarah Schwartz, "Viva Vagus: Wandering Nerve Could Lead to Range of Therapies," *Science News*, November 13, 2015, https://www.sciencenews.org/article/viva-vagus-wandering-nerve-could-lead-range-therapies (accessed May 7, 2016).

12. "FAQ: NeuroPace Responsive Neurostimulation for Epilepsy," UCSF.edu, last updated May 4, 2016, http://neurosurgery.ucsf.edu/index.php/clinical_programs_epilepsy_neuro stimulation_FAQ.html (accessed May 7, 2016).

a. Anna Hodgekiss, "Teenager's Epilepsy Is 'Cured' Thanks to Robot That Creates Sat-Nav of the Brain and Locates Exact Spot Triggering the Seizures," *Daily Mail*, February 2, 2016, http://www.dailymail.co.uk/health/article-3427985/Teenager-s-epilepsy-cured-thanks -robot-creates-sat-nav-brain-locates-exact-spot-triggering-seizures.html (accessed May 7, 2016).
b. Andrew Smith, *100 Sideways Miles* (New York: Simon & Schuster, 2014), p. 13.
c. Smith, *100 Sideways Miles*, p. 26.
d. Smith, *100 Sideways Miles*, pp. 8–9.

# Chapter 6

1. Gillian Mangan, "An Elegy to Epilepsy," *Gillian's Journey* (blog), March 22, 2016, http:// findingfaces.weebly.com/blog/an-elegy-for-epilepsy#comments (accessed June 4, 2016).
2. Samantha Jarvis, "Samantha's Story," CureEpilepsy.org, n.d., http://www.cureepilepsy.org/ share/my-story.asp?story=162 (accessed May 14, 2016).
3. See Gillian Mangan, "The Faces Project: What Is It?" FindingFaces.Weebly.com, n.d., http:// findingfaces.weebly.com/the-faces-project (accessed June 2, 2016).
4. Gillian Mangan, "Unexpected Encounters and Updates," *Gillian's Journey* (blog), November 20, 2015, http://findingfaces.weebly.com/blog/unexpected-encounters-updates (accessed June 2, 2016).
5. Mangan, "An Elegy to Epilepsy."
6. See Epilepsy Foundation, "Seizure Dogs," Epilepsy.com, n.d., http://www.epilepsy.com/get -help/staying-safe/seizure-dogs (accessed May 12, 2016).
7. See "Seizure Alert Dog," YouTube video, posted by Corrie Felder, January 29, 2016, https://www.youtube.com/watch?v=6nKvFnmvOiM and https://www.youtube.com/ watch?v=fKP5Krvq6sg (accessed May 12, 2016).
8. "Teen with Epilepsy Warns of Serious Consequences When Strangers Pet Service Dogs without Permission," Reshareworthy.com, n.d., http://www.reshareworthy.com/stranger -pets-service-dog-of-teen-with-epilepsy/ (accessed June 18, 2016).
9. See "Partner with a Dog," K94Life.org, n.d., http://k94life.org/programs/servicedog/ (accessed May 13, 2016).
10. Natalie Gross, "Dog Helps Teen Girl with Epilepsy Complete High School Education," *Lubbock Avalanche-Journal*, June 9, 2014, http://www.yourhoustonnews.com/courier/news/ dog-helps-teen-girl-with-epilepsy-complete-high-school-education/article_fa5ac9b6-9179 -56cd-9e7f-26cdd6cc0d47.html (accessed June 7, 2016).
11. Beth Galvin, "Seizure Response Dog Gives Young Georgia Woman Hope, Independence," *Fox 5 News*, May 6, 2016, updated May 9, 2016, http://www.fox5atlanta.com/health/fox -medical-team/138096023-story (accessed May 12, 2016).
12. Donna Olmsted, "Teen with Epilepsy Finds Safety with Service Dog," *Albuquerque Journal*, March 31, 2014, http://www.abqjournal.com/376234/teen-with-epilepsy-finds-safety-with -service-dog.html (accessed May 12, 2016).
13. Olmstead, "Teen with Epilepsy Finds Safety."

## Chapter 7

1. Kayla Brown, "My WebMD: A Teen Copes with Epilepsy," WebMD.com, n.d., http://www.webmd.com/epilepsy/features/teen-copes-with-epilepsy (accessed June 15, 2016).
2. See the booklet by Abbott Laboratories, *Straight Talk on Epilepsy: What Kids Need to Know* (Abbott Park, IL: Abbott Laboratories, 2006), p. 4. http://www.bcepilepsy.com/files/Information_Sheets/Straight_Talk_on_Epilepsy_What_Kids_Need_to_Know.pdf (accessed May 17, 2016).
3. "Epilepsy: Gemma—Interview 20," HealthTalk.org, n.d., http://www.healthtalk.org/young-peoples-experiences/epilepsy/gemma-interview-20 (accessed June 15, 2016).
4. "Epilepsy: Gemma—Interview 20."
5. "Epilepsy: Gemma—Interview 20."
6. Kelsie Passolt, "Epileptic Teen's Seizures at School Stop in Non-Traditional Setting," WREX.com, January 13, 2016, www.wrex.com/story/30951403/2016/01/13/epileptic-teens-seizures-at-school-stop-in-non-traditional-setting (accessed April 23, 2016).
7. Passolt, "Epileptic Teen's Seizures."
8. U.S. Equal Employment Opportunity Commission, "Questions & Answers about Epilepsy in the Workplace and the Americans with Disabilities Act (ADA)," EEOC.gov, n.d., https://www.eeoc.gov/laws/types/epilepsy.cfm (accessed May 15, 2016).
9. Samantha Jarvis, "Samantha's Story," CureEpilepsy.org, n.d., http://www.cureepilepsy.org/share/my-story.asp?story=162 (accessed May 6, 2016).
10. Strugglingtochasemydreams, "Epilepsy and Dream Job," Community Forum on Epilepsy.com, June 21, 2016, https://www.epilepsy.com/connect/forums/teens-speak/epilepsy-and-dream-job (accessed September 21, 2016).
11. Peter Fox, "Dating: The Big Dilemma," Epilepsy.org.uk, February 13, 2015, https://www.epilepsy.org.uk/news/features/dating-big-dilemma-63773 (accessed May 16, 2016).
12. Helen, interview on the "Dating, Relationships and Sex" page, HealthTalk.org, http://www.healthtalk.org/young-peoples-experiences/epilepsy/dating-relationships-and-sex (accessed May 16, 2016); note: click on "Show Text Version" under the video with Helen's name.
13. Finlay, interview on the "Dating, Relationships and Sex" page, HealthTalk.org, http://www.healthtalk.org/young-peoples-experiences/epilepsy/dating-relationships-and-sex#ixzz48pF8naEb (accessed May 16, 2016); note: click on "Show Text Version" under the video with Finlay's name.

---

a. Phylis Feiner Johnson, "Epilepsy Bill of Rights," EpilepsyTalk.com, November 5, 2015, https://epilepsytalk.com/2015/11/05/epilepsy-bill-of-rights-3/ (accessed May 13, 2016).
b. "Epilepsy 101," GirlswithNerve.com, August 2015, http://girlswithnerve.com/epilepsy-101/ (accessed May 17, 2016).

## Chapter 8

1. Josh Bean, "Boo Simon Walks Away from Football after Being Diagnosed with Epilepsy," AL.com, March 26, 2012, http://www.al.com/sports/index.ssf/2012/03/boo_simon_walks_away_from_foot.html (accessed June 15, 2016).
2. Elaine Syllie, MD, "Epilepsy Experiences—Outstanding Athlete Gets Back in the Game," *U.S. News and World Report*, November 13, 2015, http://health.usnews.com/health-news/

patient-advice/articles/2015/11/13/epilepsy-experiences-outstanding-athlete-gets-back-in
-the-game (accessed May 21, 2016).

3. Syllie, "Epilepsy Experiences."

4. Bean, "Boo Simon Walks Away from Football."

5. Sue Mott, "You Don't Have to Be an Olympic Athlete to Conquer Epilepsy—But It Certainly Helps," *Daily Mail*, March 12, 2011, http://www.dailymail.co.uk/health/article
-1365565/You-dont-Olympic-athlete-conquer-epilepsy-certainly-helps.html (accessed May 22, 2016)

6. Epilepsy Foundation, "Epilepsy Camps," Epilepsy.com, 2016, http://www.epilepsy.com/get
-help/services-and-support/camps/epilepsy-camps (accessed May 18, 2016). All of the quotes in this section come from the Epilepsy Foundation website.

7. Robert S. Fisher, MD, "Epilepsy and Recreation Safety," HealthGuru.com, January 17, 2014, http://conditions.healthguru.com/video/epilepsy-and-recreation-safety (accessed May 19, 2016).

8. Steven C. Schachter, MD, Patricia O. Shafer, RN, and Joseph I. Sirven, MD, "Safety with Exercise and Sports," adapted from *Brainstorms Companion: Epilepsy in Our View, Living Safely with Epilepsy*, September 2013, http://www.epilepsy.com/get-help/staying-safe/safety
-exercise-and-sports (accessed May 19, 2016).

a. Dayton Children's, "'I Have Epilepsy; It Doesn't Have Me,'" *Growing Together*, Summer 2012, p. 4, http://www.childrensdayton.org/cms/resource_library/files/5d73d31c2f06bafa/gtsummer12final.pdf (accessed May 22, 2016).

b. Robert Skead and Mike Simmel, *Mighty Mike Bounces Back: A Boy's Life with Epilepsy* (Washington, DC: Magination Press, 2011), p. 67.

c. Austin Aslan, *The Islands at the End of the World* (New York: Wendy Lamb/Random House, 2014), p. 6.

d. Aslan, *The Islands at the End of the World*, p. 40.

# Chapter 9

1. Dani, "Getting the Word Out," GirlswithNerve.com, August 29, 2015, http://girlswithnerve
.com/danis-letter/ (accessed June 15, 2016).

2. "Epilepsy and Women," reviewed by Richard Senelick, MD, WebMD.com, July 15, 2014, http://www.webmd.com/epilepsy/womens-issues-epilepsy (accessed May 23, 2016).

3. Amanda, "Being Diagnosed," GirlswithNerve.com, August 29, 2015, http://girlswithnerve
.com/being-diagnosed/ (accessed June 15, 2016).

4. See "Contraception, Fertility and Pregnancy," HealthTalk.org, last updated March 2014, http://www.healthtalk.org/young-peoples-experiences/epilepsy/contraception-fertility-and
-pregnancy (accessed June 9, 2016).

5. See "Contraception, Fertility and Pregnancy."

6. Heather Yade Girardin, "Epilepsy Stories," EpilepsyStories.com, 2015, http://www
.epilepsystories.com/heathers-story/ (accessed May 24, 2016).

7. Elana Gartner, "My Fears about Being a Mom with Epilepsy," kveller.com, February 28, 2013, http://www.kveller.com/my-fears-about-being-a-mom-with-epilepsy/ (accessed May 27, 2016).

8. Gartner, "My Fears about Being a Mom with Epilepsy."

9. Gartner, "My Fears about Being a Mom with Epilepsy."

10. "Epilepsy and Your Changing Hormones," reviewed by Neil Lava, MD, WebMD.com, July 20, 2014, http://www.webmd.com/epilepsy/guide/your-changing-hormones#1 (accessed May 24, 2016).

11. "Epilepsy and Your Changing Hormones."

12. Jane G. Boggs, MD, and Selim R. Benbadis, MD, "Women's Health and Epilepsy," Medscape .com, November 30, 2014, http://emedicine.medscape.com/article/1186482-overview#a3 (accessed May 25, 2016).

13. Jeff Evans, "Women with Epilepsy Conceive at Normal Rate," *Clinical Neurology News*, April 19, 2016, http://www.clinicalneurologynews.com/specialty-focus/epilepsy-seizures/single -article-page/women-with-epilepsy-conceive-at-normal-rate/b87d79eeb5d17cd851bdb6fb 1f0c9b6e.html (accessed May 26, 2016).

14. Evans, "Women with Epilepsy Conceive at Normal Rate."

a. See Kristin Seaborg, "About," *One in Twenty-Six* (blog), n.d., https://oneintwentysix.com/ about/ (accessed June 14, 2016).

b. Kristin Seaborg, "My Story," *One in Twenty-Six* (blog), October 21, 2012, https://onein twentysix.com/2012/10/21/my-story/ (accessed June 14, 2016).

c. Kristin Seaborg, "Book Excerpt! From *The Sacred Disease: A Memoir of Life with Epilepsy*," *One in Twenty-Six* (blog), June 10, 2015, https://oneintwentysix.com/2015/06/10/ book-excerpt-from-the-sacred-disease-a-memoir-of-life-with-epilepsy/?blogsub=confirmin g#blog_subscription-2. Also Kristin Seaborg, MD, *The Sacred Disease: My Life with Epilepsy* (Amazon self-published paperback, 2015), p. 199.

# Chapter 10

1. Hayden Panettiere, "Hayden Panettiere on Empowering Others with Epilepsy," video on TalkaboutIt.org, n.d., http://talkaboutit.org/hayden-panettiere-empowering-others-epilepsy (accessed June 15, 2016).

2. Harrison Ford, "Harrison Ford Wants You to Talk about Epilepsy!" video on TalkaboutIt .org, 2016, http://talkaboutit.org/harrison-ford-wants-you-talk-about-it (accessed September 20, 2016).

3. See the first edition of *Epilepsy: The Ultimate Teen Guide* (Lanham, MD: Scarecrow Press, 2002), p. 47.

4. See "How It Affects Your Family," HealthTalk.org, n.d., www.healthtalk.org/peoples -experiences/nerves-brain/epilepsy/how-it-affects-your-family (accessed June 1, 2016).

5. See "How It Affects Your Family."

6. Samme Kent, personal interview with the author, June 10, 2016.

7. Mary Jane England, Catharyn T. Liverman, Andrea M. Schultz, and Larisa M. Strawbridge, editors, *Epilepsy across the Spectrum: Promoting Health and Understanding* (Washington, DC: National Academies Press, 2012), p. 328.

8. Tom Stanton, "The Impact of SUDEP: A Message for Families Living with Epilepsy," SmartMonitor.com, www.somointeractive.com/smartmonitor/the-impact-of-sudep-a -message-for-families-living-with-epilepsy/ (accessed September 20, 2016).

9. Jaimee Bartlett, "Kimberly," sudepglobalconversation.com, February 2016, www.sudep globalconversation.com/#!kimberly/c1o15 (accessed June 1, 2016).

a. Mollie Guthrey, "For Rosemount Father and Son, Epilepsy Is a Family Story," *Pioneer Press*, November 13, 2015, http://www.twincities.com/2015/11/13/for-rosemount-father-and-son -epilepsy-is-a-family-story/ (accessed January 14, 2016).

b. Allen Costantini, "Father, Son Thankful for Kill's Epilepsy Support," *Florida Today*, October 28, 2015, http://www.floridatoday.com/story/news/2015/10/28/father-son-thankful-kills -epilepsy-support/74763012/ (accessed May 31, 2016).

# Chapter 11

1. Andy Nguyen, "Don't Let It Hold You Back," CureEpilepsy.org, n.d., http://www.cure epilepsy.org/share/my-story.asp?story=176 (accessed June 3, 2016).

2. Nguyen, "Don't Let It Hold You Back."

3. "Has Epilepsy Forced You to Change Your Career Goals?" EpilepsyFoundation.ning.com, May 5, 2013, http://epilepsyfoundation.ning.com/forum/topics/has-epilepsy-forced-you-to -change-your-career-goals (accessed June 15, 2016).

4. "Epilepsy," Reddit.com, n.d., https://www.reddit.com/r/Epilepsy/comments/1w7nip/ joining_the_army_as_ex_epilepsy_patient/ (accessed June 10, 2016).

5. See Phil, "New to Epilepsy.com," Community Forum on Epilepsy.com, n.d., http://www .epilepsy.com/connect/forums/new-epilepsycom/new-epilepticepilepsy-and-military-0 (accessed September 20, 2016).

6. Philip, "New to Epileptic/Epilepsy and the Military," n.d., posted to Epilepsy.com community forum, Epilepsy.com, http://www.epilepsy.com/connect/forums/new-epilepsycom/ new-epilepticepilepsy-and-military-0 (accessed June 5, 2016).

7. Philip, "New to Epileptic/Epilepsy and the Military."

8. SPC Allyson, "Army Will Not Give Me a Medical Discharge for Seizures," n.d., posted to Veterans with Seizures community forum, Epilepsy.com, http://www.epilepsy.com/connect/ forums/veterans-seizures/army-will-not-give-me-medical-discharge-seizures (accessed July 19, 2016).

9. See http://benefits.va.gov/BENEFITS/factsheets/general/PEBFactSheet.pdf; also see http:// www.benefits.va.gov/BENEFITS/benefits-summary/SummaryofVANationalGuardand Reserve.pdf (accessed June 6, 2016).

10. See *SEIZED: Inside the Mystery of Epilepsy*, http://www.pbs.org/program/seized-inside -mystery-epilepsy/ (accessed June 13, 2016).

11. *Tacoma News Tribune*, "Vets Face Epilepsy as Side Effect of Head Trauma," Military. com, October 26, 2013, http://www.military.com/daily-news/2013/10/26/war-veterans-face -epilepsy-as-side-effect-of-head-trauma.html (accessed June 3, 2016).

12. Colby Strong, ed. "Is PTSD a Precursor to Psychogenic Nonepileptic Seizures in Veterans?" *Neurology Review*, June 21, 2013, http://www.neurologyreviews.com/specialty-focus/ epilepsy/article/is-ptsd-a-precursor-to-psychogenic-nonepileptic-seizures-in-veterans/5e30 00b67be7299c6a30954949ec6bd7.html (accessed June 6, 2016).

13. Annette M. Boyle, "Then, and Now: VA Innovates in Epilepsy Treatment and Evaluation," USMedicine.com, November 2014, http://www.usmedicine.com/agencies/department-of -veterans-affairs/then-and-now-va-innovates-in-epilepsy-treatment-and-evaluation/ (accessed July 19, 2016).

14. Boyle, "Then and Now."

15. Veterans Administration, "VA Epilepsy Center of Excellence Releases Video Series on Veterans with Epilepsy," Epilepsy.com, February 2016, http://www.epilepsy.com/article/2016/2/va-epilepsy-center-excellence-releases-video-series-veterans-epilepsy (accessed June 2, 2016).

16. Veterans Administration, "VA Epilepsy Center of Excellence Releases Video Series."

a. U.S. Department of Defense. *Medical Standards for Appointment, Enlistment, or Induction in the Military Services*, 2010, http://www.dtic.mil/whs/directives/corres/pdf/613003p.pdf (accessed July 19, 2016).

b. Blake Stilwell, "Here's Why Most Americans Can't Join the Military," *Business Insider*, September 28, 2015, http://www.businessinsider.com/heres-why-most-americans-cant-join-the-military-2015-9 (accessed June 6, 2016).

c. "Exceptional Family Member Program Facts," crdamc.amedd.army.mil, August 2014, http://www.crdamc.amedd.army.mil/efmp/facts.aspx (accessed June 13, 2016).

# Chapter 12

1. Jason Jordan, "Kathryn Stevens Takes the Capitol," *Evening Tribune*, April 26, 2016, http://www.eveningtribune.com/article/20160426/NEWS/160429792 (accessed June 12, 2016).

2. CNN Wire, "Teen Collapses, Suffers Seizure during First Beauty Pageant," Fox59.com, May 9, 2016, http://fox59.com/2016/05/09/teen-collapses-suffers-seizure-during-first-beauty-pageant/ (accessed May 27, 2016).

3. CNN Wire, "Teen Collapses, Suffers Seizure during First Beauty Pageant."

4. Rebecca Croomes, "Area Teen Advocates Epilepsy Awareness," *News Courier*, October 22, 2014, http://www.enewscourier.com/news/local_news/area-teen-advocates-epilepsy-awareness/article_dc2a10d2-5972-11e4-8930-bf42c52ef149.html (accessed June 5, 2016).

5. Sharon Roznik, "Friends Help Fond du Lac Teen Battle Epilepsy," *Fond du Lac Reporter*, April 8, 2015, www.fdlreporter.com/story/news/local/2015/04/08/micolichek-epilepsy/25479363/ (accessed September 20, 2016).

6. Jordan, "Kathryn Stevens Takes the Capitol."

7. See http://www.epilepsygroup.com/news6-85/bike-a-thon-to-raise-awareness-on-epilepsy-and-seizure.htm (accessed May 19, 2016).

8. See the FACES website at http://faces.med.nyu.edu/ (accessed June 2, 2016).

9. See National Institute of Neurological Disorders and Stroke, *Hope through Research* (Bethesda, MD: National Institute of Health, 2015), https://catalog.ninds.nih.gov/pubstatic//15-156/15-156.pdf (accessed June 10, 2016).

10. "Alternative Treatments for Epilepsy," reviewed by Richard Senelick, MD, WebMD.com, July 14, 2014, http://www.webmd.com/epilepsy/guide/are-there-alternative-treatments (accessed June 7, 2016).

11. National Institute of Neurological Disorders and Stroke, "NINDS Epilepsy Information Page," NINDS.NIH.gov, February 1, 2016, http://www.ninds.nih.gov/disorders/epilepsy/epilepsy.htm (accessed June 10, 2016).

12. See Ian, "Ian's Story," Neuropace.com, n.d., http://www.neuropace.com/ians-story/ (accessed June 13, 2016).

13. Citizens United for Research in Epilepsy, *State of Research in the Epilepsies 2013* (Chicago: CURE, 2013), p. 4, available at http://www.cureepilepsy.org/downloads/research/state-of-epilepsy.pdf (accessed September 21, 2016).

14. Robert Preidt, "One-a-Day Anti-Seizure Drug Shows Promise for People with Epilepsy," HealthDay.com, April 14, 2016, https://consumer.healthday.com/cognitive-health-information-26/epilepsy-news-235/one-a-day-anti-seizure-drug-looks-promising-709832.html (accessed September 21, 2016).

15. "Neural Stem Cell Implants Hold Promise for Treating Epilepsy, Says UF Researchers," *Space Coast Daily*, May 4, 2015, http://spacecoastdaily.com/2015/05/neural-stem-cell-implants-hold-promise-for-treating-epilepsy-says-uf-researchers/ (accessed May 28, 2016).

16. Louisiana State University Health Sciences Center, "Novel Compound Switches Off Epilepsy Development," *Science Daily*, January 28, 2015, https://www.sciencedaily.com/releases/2015/01/150128113830.htm (accessed June 15, 2016).

17. Susan Barber Lindquist, "Data from Dogs and People Advances Epileptic Seizure Forecasting," MayoClinic.org, May 24, 2016, http://newsnetwork.mayoclinic.org/discussion/crowdsourcing-contest-using-data-from-people-dogs-advances-epileptic-seizure-forecasting/ (accessed September 20, 2016).

18. Mayo Clinic, "Crowdsourcing Contest Using Data from People, Dogs Advances Epileptic Seizure Forecasting," *Science Daily*, May 24, 2016, https://www.sciencedaily.com/releases/2016/05/160524144917.htm (accessed June 17, 2016).

19. Anne Brown, "New Studies Highlight Potential Genetic Factors Underlying SUDEP," EpilepsyResearch.org.uk, December 11, 2015, https://www.epilepsyresearch.org.uk/new-studies-highlight-potential-genetic-factors-underlying-sudep/ (accessed June 8, 2016).

a. See "Humour and Jokes about Epilepsy," HealthTalk.org, n.d., http://www.healthtalk.org/young-peoples-experiences/epilepsy/humour-and-jokes-about-epilepsy (accessed June 9, 2016).

# Glossary

**absence seizure**: a generalized seizure characterized by staring or twitching and jerking of muscles.

**antiepileptic drug (AED)**: a drug used to treat the chronic condition of epilepsy.

**atonic seizure**: a seizure causing a sudden loss of muscle tone.

**aura**: a small partial seizure that causes unusual sensations and acts as a warning that a larger seizure is about to occur.

**axon**: long, fiber-like part of a neuron by which the cell sends information to receiving neurons.

**cell body**: contains the nucleus and cytoplasm of a cell.

**cell membrane**: boundary separating the inside contents of a cell from its surrounding environment.

**clonic seizure**: an epileptic seizure characterized by jerking.

**complex partial seizure**: a seizure that begins in a specific location in the brain that alters consciousness or causes loss of consciousness.

**computerized axial tomography (CAT or CT)**: a computer scan that creates X-ray with detailed images of the brain.

**convulsion**: stiffening of the body and jerking.

**dendrite**: point of contact for receiving impulses on a neuron, branching off from the cell body.

**dopamine**: a neurotransmitter mainly involved in controlling movement, managing the release of various hormones, and aiding the flow of information to the front of the brain.

**drop attack**: another term for an atonic seizure.

**electrode**: a small metal contact attached to a wire designed to record brain waves from the scalp or inside the brain.

**electroencephalogram (EEG)**: a test that traces brain waves with electrodes.

**epileptologist**: a neurologist who specializes in epilepsy treatment.

**fit**: an outdated and inaccurate term for a seizure.

**gene**: segment of DNA that codes to make proteins and other important body chemicals.

**generalized seizure**: a seizure that affects many parts of the brain.

**grand mal seizure**: an older term for a tonic-clonic seizure.

**hippocampus**: portion of the brain involved in creating and filing new memories.

**intractable seizure**: a seizure that cannot be stopped by medication.

**intrauterine device (IUD):** a small, flexible plastic device inserted into a woman's uterus to prevent pregnancy.

**magnetic resonance imaging (MRI):** a scan that uses a large magnet instead of X-rays to form a detailed image of the brain.

**neuron:** a nerve cell.

**neurotransmitter:** chemical produced by neurons that carries messages to other neurons.

**nucleus:** structure within a cell that contains DNA and information the cell needs for growing, staying alive, and making new neurons.

**partial seizure:** a seizure that begins in a specific location in the brain, such as the temporal lobe.

**petit mal seizure:** an older term for an absence seizure.

**simple partial seizure:** a seizure that begins in a specific location in the brain and produces an abnormal sensation.

**synapse:** tiny gap between neurons, where nerve impulses are sent from one neuron to another.

**temporal lobe:** a part of the brain important in memory and controlling speech.

**tonic seizure:** a seizure that causes muscles to stiffen.

**vagus nerve stimulator (VNS):** a device implanted in the upper chest, which stimulates a nerve that can reduce seizure activity.

# Further Resources

## Books

Bogash, James. *Migraines and Epilepsy: How to Find Relief, Live Well, and Protect Your Brain* (New York: Morgan James Publishing, 2015).

Jines-Burritt, Lola. *Epilepsy Unveiled: Caretaking, Seizures, Psychosis and Brain Surgery* (Sanford, TX: BLB Publishing, 2012).

Kossoff, Eric, John M. Freeman, Zahava Turner, and James E. Rubenstein. *Ketogenic Diets: Treatments for Epilepsy and Other Disorders*, 5th ed. (New York: Demos Health, 2011).

National Institute of Neurological Disorders and Stroke, National Institutes of Health. *The Epilepsies and Seizures: Hope Through Research* (Bethesda, MD: National Institute of Neurological Disorders and Stroke National Institutes of Health, 2015).

Sazgar, Mona and Cynthia L. Harden, MD., eds. *Controversies in Caring for Women with Epilepsy*. (Switzerland: Springer International Publishing, 2016)

Seaborg, Kristin. *The Sacred Disease: My Life with Epilepsy*, 2nd ed. (Kristin-SeaborgBooks, 2016).

## Websites

4 Paws for Ability: http://4pawsforability.org/

Canine Partners for Life: http://k94life.org/programs/servicedog/

The Charlie Foundation for Ketogenic Therapies: www.charliefoundation.org

Citizens United for Research in Epilepsy (CURE): www.cureepilepsy.org

Clinical Neurology News: www.clinicalneurologynews.com

Epilepsy Foundation: www.epilepsy.com

Epilepsy Museum in Kork: http://www.epilepsiemuseum.de/alt/body_diagnostiken.html

Epilepsy Stories: http://www.epilepsystories.com/

Living Well with Epilepsy: www.livingwellwithepilepsy.com

Paws with a Cause: https://www.pawswithacause.org/what-we-do/seizure-dogs

Service Dogs for America: http://www.servicedogsforamerica.org/about-us/service-dogs/emergency-medical-response-dogs/

WebMD Epilepsy Help Center: http://www.webmd.com/epilepsy/default.htm

# Index

# About the Author

**Kathlyn Gay** is the author of more than 120 nonfiction books for children, teenagers, and adults. Her work focuses on diverse subjects, including social, environmental and multicultural issues, and history. She has done extensive research on numerous topics for her wide variety of books, which reviewers call "factual, well-organized, straightforward, and readable." Gay has also authored/edited several encyclopedias. She is the author of a number of titles in the It Happened to Me series:

- *Activism: The Ultimate Teen Guide* (2016)
- *Divorce: The Ultimate Teen Guide* (2014)
- *Bigotry and Intolerance: The Ultimate Teen Guide* (2013)
- *Living Green: The Ultimate Teen Guide* (2012)
- *Body Image and Appearance: The Ultimate Teen Guide* (2009)
- *The Military and Teens: The Ultimate Teen Guide* (2008)
- *Religion and Spirituality in America: The Ultimate Teen Guide* (2006)
- *Volunteering: The Ultimate Teen Guide* (2004)
- *Cultural Diversity: The Ultimate Teen Guide* (2003)